Reflection for Nursing Life

Over the past decades, reflection has taken centre stage in nursing education. However, it is easy to get stuck in a superficial cycle of storytelling and self-examination without getting any further insights into your own practice and abilities. *Reflection for Nursing Life* starts with a basic introduction to reflective practice and moves on to look at more critical perspectives, with guidance for reflecting on the complex realities of practice.

This accessible text is designed to support a deeper understanding of the value of reflection and its relationship with the needs of modern practice. Beginning with discussions of self-awareness and the reflective cycle, the book goes on to explore ideas about critical incidents, critical reflection models and transformational learning. It integrates cutting-edge neuro-scientific research and thinking about emotional labour and intelligence in healthcare into mainstream reflective practice, drawing on both new and established ways of guiding learning and professional judgment.

Reflection for Nursing Life includes numerous exemplar reflective narratives, diagrams and exercises to help the reader identify their strengths and weaknesses, whilst tips for overcoming weaknesses and developing strengths are also provided. This is the ideal text for nursing students and practitioners looking to improve their reflective practice skills.

John McKinnon is a Senior Lecturer in Nursing at the University of Lincoln, UK. He was a front-line practitioner for 20 years and has researched, taught and published on reflective practice and emotional intelligence which were the focus of his doctorate.

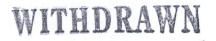

'John McKinnon's text is a comprehensive and highly readable exploration of the area. The use of stories enables the reader to consider their own practice and will appeal to a variety of health care professionals. The focus on resilience, humanity and engagement is both powerful and refreshing.'

Carolyn Crouchman, *Senior Lecturer, Advanced Health Care,*
Buckinghamshire New University, UK

'Written with a strong blend of the theoretical and the practical, this book is an excellent resource for those who wish to enhance their reflective skills whilst understanding more fully the theoretical underpinning of such skills. Written in a learned but accessible manner, interspersed with anecdotes and stories, the book is useful to students, novices and more experienced staff. One of the strengths of the book is its early focus on the understanding of self as a foundation of effective practice, often a step in the reflective journey that is omitted in other texts. The opening chapter of McKinnon's book emphasises the importance of self-awareness in becoming an effective reflector and acknowledges the importance of acknowledging one's own humanity. This important fact is a theme throughout the book, as is the necessity of a sense of self when undertaking reflective activity.

The book is distinct from many of the the other reflective texts in that it focuses on reflection in nursing life, acknowledging that one may still be a nurse, even when one is not actually 'doing nursing' and these periods are often the times when reflection can take place. McKinnon's approach to reflection is based upon principles, rather than on process, highlighting the belief that it should be part of everything nurses are, rather than another task to be completed.

I found this to be an extremely edifying book, which made me look at my practice and myself in a different way. Practitioners, educators and researchers will find this book a useful source of inspiration and information.'

Professor Carol Haigh, *Faculty Health, Psychology & Social Care,*
Manchester Metropolitan University, UK

'Reflective practice is an essential part of nursing life and supports personal and professional development. John McKinnon's thought-provoking and practical book offers new ways of thinking about this well-known concept. The use of practitioner narratives enhance the text and bring the associated theory to life. This book will support all health care professionals who want to develop their reflective thinking.'

Dr Kirsten Jack, *Senior Lecturer in Adult Nursing,*
Manchester Metropolitan University, UK

Reflection for Nursing Life

Principles, process and practice

John McKinnon

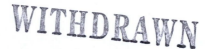
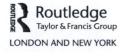

Routledge
Taylor & Francis Group

LONDON AND NEW YORK

KH

First published 2016
by Routledge
2 Park Square, Milton Park, Abingdon, Oxon OX14 4RN

and by Routledge
711 Third Avenue, New York, NY 10017

Routledge is an imprint of the Taylor & Francis Group, an informa business

© 2016 J. McKinnon

British Library Cataloguing in Publication Data
A catalogue record for this book is available from the British Library

Library of Congress Cataloging in Publication Data
A catalogue record for this book has been requested.

ISBN: 978-1-138-78758-2 (hbk)
ISBN: 978-1-138-78759-9 (pbk)
ISBN: 978-1-315-76632-4 (ebk)

Typeset in Times New Roman
by Swales & Willis Ltd, Exeter, Devon, UK

10/18/17

Dedicated to Jon Robert, the son I always wished for.
From Dad.

Contents

Figures

Tables

Boxes

Foreword

John McKinnon's book offers a new and exciting perspective on nurses' professionalism. This is in stark contrast to the picture we have of nursing that we inherited from the 19th and early part of the 20th century, where the ideal model was that of detachment, compliance to the dictates of the expert (usually a male doctor), a fixed rather than changing view of how to behave, relatively low levels of education and training and above all a non-reflective view of the profession. Indeed, it was only with the greatest of difficulty that one could have called nursing a profession.

There are three models of nursing: craft, technician and professional. Craft knowledge has the following characteristics. It is rooted in practice and this rules out certain types of learning approaches. This means that imitation and scaffolding various attempts to perform the activities are key to the development of this type of knowledge. The teacher or facilitator is the expert practitioner and knowledge is derived from exposure to the performances of the expert. The expert is therefore not a skilled pedagogue but a skilled practitioner. The emphasis is on observing and imitating the practice. The justification for this is that the nature of the practice is better understood in these terms, that is, the learning object, becoming and being a good nurse, are craft activities.

The second of our models is the executive technician. This requires the nurse to perform in a particular way; to have, and be able to execute, a repertoire of pre-conceived actions. This is a rule-based activity and learning is understood as the assimilation of these rules and ways of enacting them, without recourse to critical reflection or situated understanding. The executive technician model recognises the value of research findings, and this means that it is not thought appropriate for nurses to interpret those findings for themselves. Nursing researchers generate findings which are then expressed as protocols for action, and the role of the nurse is to implement these protocols in the most efficient way they can. One consequence of this is that the knowledge which is being transferred lacks a sense of change, emergence, immediacy or relevance. This positions the learning object, these rules and protocols, outside space and time and effectively reifies it. The rules they follow are therefore not situation-specific or even sensitive to the particularities of the setting in which they are being applied.

Both of these can be contrasted with professional learning. Professional learning emanates and is derived from an understanding of the characteristics and functions of becoming and being a nurse. Apart from the content and methodological knowledge that nurses need in order to function, they also have to take a variety of other factors into consideration and integrate them in a coherent, efficient and effective way. But above all, they have to act therapeutically, and accept that emotional attachment is the key to successful performance. This is the gist of the argument that John McKinnon makes in this book, and it is radical and emancipatory. It understands nursing as emotionally charged, meta-reflective, a professional learning experience and above all a caring profession.

Professor David Scott
University College London, Institute of Education,
University of London

Introduction

The reader who finds this book on a shelf or on an electronic device may well ask whether nursing needs yet another book on reflection. My answer is a resounding 'Yes!'. This book arises in part out of my dissatisfaction with existing texts. However, my chief motivation was my frustration with the large number of undergraduate and postgraduate learners who continue to struggle with what is an important key to independent thinking and learning in order to steer professional development. My main goal in producing the book is essentially to present the subject of reflection in a way which breaks down barriers to understanding and competence by discussing ways in which we already use the skill in our daily lives without really thinking about it. Furthermore, it should be clear from the title that the book is unashamedly aimed exclusively at the nursing profession. This is not because I choose to ignore the sweeping changes which have been taking place in health and social care such as inter-professional learning and working. Rather the book is aimed at nurses because of the characteristics and changes in recent years many of which are unique to the profession and warrant a learning text which is tailored to take account of the needs arising from these. There are a number of areas which need to be considered when attempting to write a book on reflection for nurses which attempts to make a difference to the way they think and behave in practice.

The changing face of the nursing work force and 'nursing life'

The book title refers to 'nursing life' rather than 'nursing' in acknowledgement of a significant contemporary feature of the nursing population. Hargreaves (2010) has noted a major change in the nursing work force. In modern times up until the last quarter of the 20th century the majority of nurses were unmarried and lived in nursing residences closely linked to the clinical area in which they worked. Historically the management of this accommodation was paternalistic and protective and reflected the tightly regimented and regulated manner in which the nursing profession was overseen. As an environment the nursing residential community existed separately from the rest of society with friendships and support networks which were readily available. Now a diverse workforce constitutes a nursing profession which lives outside hospital premises in the community along with the patient groups it serves. The number of mature students entering the profession has increased. Nurses are no longer solely dedicated to their work. In addition to being professional practitioners, nurses are also parents, partners and children with other responsibilities aside from those which relate to working life. There are certainly a number of advantages to this change in professional membership. A diverse workforce brings a diverse understanding to practice borne of complex life experience. As this book will show even teenage students bring much richer life experience to their study and life skills to their practice than did students of their age 40 or 50 years ago. Nurses already prepared with informal life learning in 'the University of Life' are equipped with empathy built on personal biography as well as imagination. This type of empathy is reflected in the comments of an experienced community nurse:

> I know for myself I thought I knew what it would feel like to be bereaved when I visited bereaved patients having done all the courses. I felt that I could empathise with them. But then when I lost my father I felt very different and so my empathy now is different, because I've got that lived experience of loss in somebody that you've cared about. So I would say that could only come from living through an experience and you can't learn that from a book. And that's made me a different person, emotionally, to go and see somebody who is bereaved.

So a diverse nursing workforce membership embedded within the fabric of a community means that the population find better representation in a nursing profession which is more attuned to public health needs. However, there are also disadvantages. For modern nurses, rich life narratives bring multiple life roles which compete with and threaten to encroach upon professional life. In addition, professional life also threatens to encroach on other life roles. This is reflected in the narrative of one experienced children's nurse who was also a forty-year-old mother of two and a carer of an aging parent:

> There's so much we're trying to squeeze into twenty-four hours that I feel sometimes there's not enough hours for me. I've got exams to read for, I'm still working my normal shifts, there's family life, kids to take care of, parents evening, shopping, domestic stuff to be done, dad to take to the doctors' and its overwhelming sometimes.

Notice from the nurse's comments another feature of modern nursing life: continuing professional development at higher education level. The striving for a work life balance is borne of competing mutually informing life roles in 21st-century nursing. An absence of attention to work life balance has been shown to result in stress arising from one role spilling over onto another negatively effecting both (Peronne and Civiletto, 2004). A modern template for reflection must own the seamlessness of nursing life; the mutual interchange of learning between life health and work together with the emotional physical and mental implications.

The changing shape of nursing practice

The title also mentions 'principles' ahead of the 'process' of reflection. This is deliberate because learners cannot be expected to engage effectively with the ubiquitous process of reflection without understanding the factors which protect or inhibit what is a fragile personal activity. The central place of the nurse–patient relationship and emotional labour in modern nursing is a preoccupation which stands in sharp contrast to the directive which dominated the larger part of 20th-century nursing practice: that emotional attachment in a therapeutic relationship is foreign to ideas of professionalism (McQueen, 2004). Mazhindu's studies (2003) suggest the rectitude of emotional detachment from patients is still preserved in nursing mythology and is supported in the following narrative excerpt by a recently qualified young nurse in an intensive care unit:

> You can't always detach yourself and I think it is important to realise you are only human and you sometimes, especially with long term or chronic patients, you do get attached to them and for whatever reason, elements of that child's or family's situation may be familiar.

It is interesting that being human is seen by the nurse as a weakness rather than strength. The major shift in ideology and focus assumes that all nurses who have long been expected to suppress their emotions and shun emotional attachment are able to adapt to a patient centred approach requiring emotional investment. But there is evidence (Mazhindu, 2003) that this is not always the case. It seems that many nurses struggle to acknowledge and manage their emotions. This has implications for the self-awareness, attention to one's own needs and the level of empathy that can be exercised toward others including patients (Eckroth-Bucher, 2010). These are all prerequisites to effective reflection. The informed use of self is a powerful skill in any caring practice, but it does not come naturally or easily to everyone. For those nurses who source emotion in their practice research (Niedenthal, Krauth-Gruber and Ric, 2006; Gray, 2009b) suggests that while emotional investment in a job role rewards with a sense of achievement it also takes its toll if employees are not rested. This is evident from the narrative of a school nurse who describes how she grasped a few precious moments of peace and solitude following a morning on which she uncovered a referred and severe case of child neglect:

> Over the Bridge near . . . I found a really quiet spot, the tide coming in, I just opened the window, the wind coming in and the sky. It wasn't sunny. It was a horrible day but it didn't really matter, just trying to find some calm in the day. I think that's really important. I don't always achieve it because there isn't always the time or space to do that, it just happened having been to this meeting, before I had to go on anywhere else, I had that half hour slot where I was able to do that.

Niedenthal, Krauth-Gruber and Ric (2006) showed that perpetual suppressing of emotions can lead to low self-esteem, depressive mood states and poor life satisfaction. Relentless emotional labour also carries a psycho somatic price with an increased incidence of hypertension, coronary heart disease and cancer (Gray, 2009). Any new text which purports to guide reflection must help the learner appreciate and build the appropriate personal capital; qualities such as honesty openness and self-awareness along with abilities such as creativity and imagination.

Reflection in the context of nurse education and practice learning

Principles for sound reflective practice do not exist solely within the individual learner but extend to the environment in which reflection takes place including the learning values at work. Boud

(2010) has explained how reflection was embraced unquestionably by nursing practitioners and academics in the 1990s with little or no consideration given to the underpinning philosophy. As a result, in keeping with the paternalistic historical roots of the profession, in many schools of nursing reflective narrative was demanded of students as part of a didactic style of teaching and the distinction between reflection and essay writing was lost. The value of time space honesty self-awareness and commitment were often forgotten. Lip service was often paid to the importance of critical analysis. Consequently, for the students of that time who are today's practitioners, reflection is simply storytelling and analysis may rarely pass the stage of considering ones feelings. This has led to reflective practice being viewed with cynicism by many practitioners and theorists who question its worth (Hargreaves, 2004). Furthermore, insufficient consideration is often given to the impact of the power relationship between teacher and student on the shape of compliant pieces of reflection produced (Cameron and Mitchell, 1993; Richardson and Maltby, 1995).

Fast accessible communication technology in the shape of email, texting and social media is now the order of the day. The lack of personal human interface common to such communication and the multiple routes of conversation that can now be conducted simultaneously mean that sufficient forethought and sufficient attention are not always paid to the content and tone of messages. Any face to face contact which is attempted often has to compete with social media engagement which takes priority. I was once bemused by a student who asked me to explain again the essence of a part of my lecture she had just attended but who began to text her friend while I attempted to provide a clearer explanation! Fast communication technology and the behaviours they mould are now deeply embedded in our culture across generations. All of this presents new challenges to space and respect for reflective thought.

The culture of evidence base

Practice founded in best evidence has become a given as well as a constant in nursing (Mulhall, 1998). Nurses are required to justify their judgement and decision making with current evidence base. So it is important that once novice reflective practitioners are accustomed to self-disclosure and storytelling (an important phase which should not be rushed) they can be helped to move on to exploring the relationship between their experience and external evidence. The latter part of the 'reflection equation' is the link between a story, critical thinking and discovery learning.

The contribution of neuroscience

Since the advent of neural imaging, neuroscience has contributed much to our understanding of learning and decision making by providing support for the pre-existing arguments of learning theorists (Schon, 1989; Miller, 1990; Bruner, 1999; Rogers, 1999; Mezirow, 2000; Illeris, 2006). A main theme in this body of work has been the coupling of emotions with cognitive activity to guide judgement and decision making (Damasio, 2000; Immordino-Yang and Damassio, 2007). The functions of the structures of the mid brain such as the amygdala, hippocampi and the prefrontal cortex all improve our understanding of how we learn (Cohen, 2006; Rose, 2006). There is a need to incorporate awareness of these neural models of understanding within our approach to reflection. These understandings help us provide justification for time and space with which to reflect on our practice.

Reflection and levels of study

Today's practising nurses are all busily engaged at some point in continuing education; some at bachelor, others at masters and still others at doctoral levels of study. There is an assumption that students at higher levels of study are more skilled in reflective practice but there is no evidence to support this view. My own teaching experience has led me to believe that there are many gifted reflective practitioners at all levels of study. However, I have also noticed that there are many other learners who despite possessing a large stock hold of knowledge struggle to extract it meaningfully from their experience. Something clearly requires redress in study programmes in which students are asked and able to understand ion exchange and acid base balance but are deemed incapable of using a model of critical reflection to good effect. It is for these reasons that I refute suggestions that separate texts on reflection are appropriate for different levels of study. The structure of the book reflects a seamless approach to reflection at any stage of study. The chapters follow a logical progressive pathway in understanding reflection and its antecedents. Regardless of their level of study the reader is not patronised but offered within each chapter a choice of depth of study with the detail of underpinning theories and philosophies discussed within figures and tables and placed strategically throughout the main body of the text. While many of these figures and tables are linked to specific parts of the main text some in keeping with adult learning are in place simply to stimulate readers thinking beyond what is explicit.

All the contributed narratives are the product of either nursing students or expert nurses. However, their narratives are in the book as exemplars of reflective practice at different levels and in different ways in different situations. They are not intended to be perfect pieces of work. They are personal statements of learning cut from the fabric of individual lives and should be critiqued as such. The reader will also note that the contents reflect a positive approach to reflection which derives learning from highlighting good and excellence in practice as much as learning grown from errors. This is a deliberate attempt to move away from a culture of negative criticism and self-deprecation which has tainted reflective practice in nursing.

The structure of the book

The book attempts to explain theoretical and philosophical terms with the progression of the text but readers should also find the glossary helpful in this respect.

Chapter 1 addresses the sensitive subject of self-awareness. Generous space is given over to impact on self-awareness of the range of emotional and cultural backgrounds which bring people to nursing together with the implications for reflective practice. In this section I also explore the repertoire of personal skills and qualities which make up the therapeutic use of self.

Chapter 2 makes deliberate reference to the 'art' of reflection with the purpose of emphasising that reflection is not a uniform or substantive subject but an organic one. As such reflectivity will vary with each individual and evolve with experience of life and understanding of learning.

Chapter 3 is a response to the critique of the viability reflection as a learning tool which is more accurately a critique of how that tool has been deployed. Removing the mask of infallibility that has often been placed on reflection as a route to learning forms part of this response. However human judgement has strengths that are absent in artificial intelligence and these will also be considered.

Chapter 4 is reserved for critical incidents (or significant events) as they have value in nursing. In addition to explaining the structure of such events I also look at the psychological and neural basis for their use in learning. In addition we will visit the importance of learning from positive as well as negative experiences.

Chapter 5 is designed to help the learner progress from storytelling and demonstration of learning to critical reflection through a wider and deeper consideration of meaning. I have often found that different students struggle with different parts of the reflection process and so I have chosen to break this down and examine the skills necessary for each part in turn. Models of reflection will be discussed here and in Chapter 6, but true to the title of the book, I value the imparting of principles of reflection over adherence to any model or framework. In short, I see the use of models of reflection as an optional means rather than an essential end.

Chapter 6 takes over where Chapter 5 leaves off by introducing the theory of transformative learning. Narratives contained within this chapter carry application of transformative learning in private as well as professional life. This is part of my attempt to demystify a part of learning theory which often baffles students.

Chapter 7 presents a new framework for reflection which harnesses emotions to inform practice. The framework is built on research into the commonality of core emotions across nursing together with the extant literature on emotion and learning.

Reflection for Nursing Life is intended to be a guide for contemporary practice life and read as a learning textbook. Beyond this however stories have a power of their own to move, to provoke new thinking and to entertain. So it is my intention that nurses will enjoy and relate to the many narratives from real lives which punctuate every chapter: comparing and contrasting them with their own and creating their own learning from this.

1 Becoming a reflective practitioner – part one

Self-awareness and the use of self

Box 1.1   Main points: Chapter 1

- Self-awareness and the effective use of self are prerequisites to sound reflective practice.
- Self-awareness is important to be able to exercise compassion and empathy.
- Self-exploration is important to identify our values, prejudices and assumptions in life along with their root causes.
- Reflexivity is the ability to use a situation as a measure for the self with a view to learning and positive change.
- Mindfulness is the maximum possible resourcing of the self 'in the present moment'.

Introduction

This opening chapter, rather than being concerned with the process and practice of reflection, lays part of the groundwork for effective engagement with reflection. We will define and explore consciousness, self-awareness and the use of self. Allied notions of mindfulness and reflexivity will also be discussed along with their relationship to desirable qualities in nursing such as empathy and compassion. We will draw on psychology, philosophy, neuroscience and learning theory to understand the importance of first possessing self-awareness and competence in the use of self before becoming reflective practitioners. Old and new narratives will be used to illustrate self-awareness, mindfulness and reflexivity. Exercises in self-awareness are contained within Tables 1.1, 1.2 and 1.3.

There are a number of factors which may work to promote or inhibit reflection in a person; five of them are personal qualities and three relate to the available environment. Two of the personal qualities: self-awareness and reflexivity within the context of the use of self are the focus of this chapter. The remaining factors will be explored in Chapter 2.

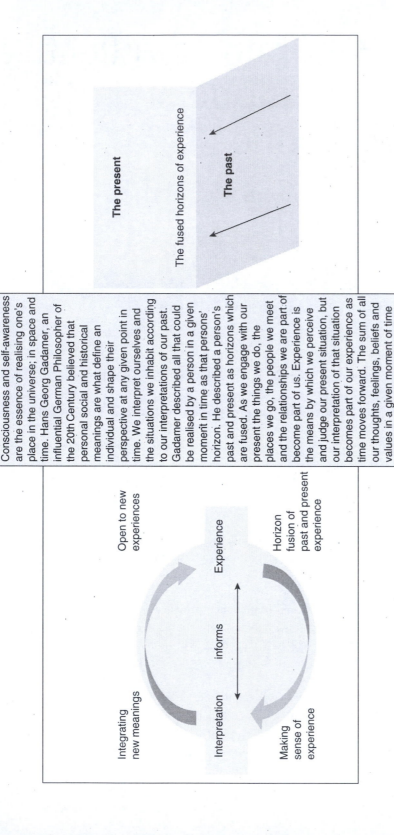

Consciousness and self-awareness are the essence of realising one's place in the universe; in space and time. Hans Georg Gadamer, an influential German Philosopher of the 20th Century believed that personal social and historical meanings are what define an individual and shape their perspective at any given point in time. We interpret ourselves and the situations we inhabit according to our interpretations of our past. Gadamer described all that could be realised by a person in a given moment in time as that persons' horizon. He described a person's past and present as horizons which are fused. As we engage with our present the things we do, the places we go, the people we meet and the relationships we are part of become part of us. Experience is the means by which we perceive and judge our present situation, but our interpretation of that situation becomes part of our experience as time moves forward. The sum of all our thoughts, feelings, beliefs and values in a given moment of time are the product of our past and present experience. Hence our fused horizon of past and present is always moving forward.

The present

The fused horizons of experience

The past

Open to new experiences

Experience

Horizon fusion of past and present experience

Integrating new meanings

informs

Interpretation

Making sense of experience

Figure 1.1 Gadamer theory

The individual as a conscious sentient being

First to become self-aware or to know ourselves we must be conscious. The term 'consciousness' is used in a very limited sense in some clinical practice settings and it can be confused with 'wakefulness'. But a person can be awake but lack conscious awareness. Extreme examples of this exist in neurological disorders but we have all known people who are remarkably unaware of their social presentation and their impact on the world around them. Consciousness in sentient beings is a sense of self; our identity in the past, present and future (Damassio, 1999). It describes our ability to define our place in space and time; to ask and strive to answer questions such as 'Who am I?', 'Where do I come from?' and 'Where am I going'. Gadamer's theory on life learning (Figure 1.1) shows how our past experience shapes how we interpret the present and ourselves as part of that experience. As time is perpetually moving forward and our experience accumulates, we are a different person today from the one we were yesterday and we become a different person tomorrow from the one we are today. This 'extended' consciousness is one of the features which separate humans from all other life on our planet (Figure 1.2). Extended consciousness is the knowing that we are who we are and that we know what we know. When we develop consciousness we begin to become self-aware. Once self-awareness is in place we are able to move forward making the most effective use of ourselves.

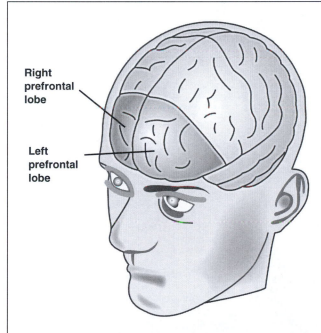

Right prefrontal lobe

Left prefrontal lobe

The enlarged prefrontal cortex (PFC) in the human brain houses extended consciousness and self-awareness. The left frontal lobe acts as an 'encoder' giving sense to information while the right lobe manages life story themes and places them in context. The medial lobe is responsible for generating confidence in judgement through a feeling of knowing. It is here, therefore, that working memory is coupled with a feeling of knowing and the decisonmaking executive (Goldberg, 2001; Modirrousta and Fellows, 2008).

Because of this we are able to experience extended consciousness with a mental image of ourselves in space and time with a past, present and future. As such our judgements and decisions reflect this awareness. The function of the prefrontal cortex and the seamless relationship between emotion and thought show the importance of self-awareness as a prerequisite to reflection. Tracing our thoughts, judgements, decisions and actions back to the emotions which accompanied them will in turn make our values and assumptions clearer to us.

Figure 1.2   Consciousness and self-awareness

Self-awareness and the use of self

The 'use of self' is the skilled sensitive shaping of one's personality and presence to achieve positive outcomes in relationships. The use of self both directs and is informed by personal learning from experience. The effective use of self begins with self-awareness arising out of a conscious knowledge of one's motives and social presentation together with how we may be perceived by others. It is the art of 'making oneself the focus of one's own attention' (Eckroth-Bucher, 2010: 300) or of developing a considered 'understanding of ourselves' (Jack and Miller, 2008: 31) in order to move effectively in the world. Table 1.1 provides a preliminary exercise in this area. Knowing oneself carries the notion of comparing one's behaviour to standards more easily applied to others; it is about discovering and seeking to close the gap between the ideal image of the self and actual reality (Eckroth-Bucher, 2010). Table 1.2 provides more help with this. Sound reflection and reflective practice rely on balanced powers of interpretation. The use of self, knowing oneself and the part one plays in situations past, present and future is essential before one can hope to interpret one's surroundings and the actions of others in a balanced way.

The concept of self-awareness is consistent with Gadamer's vision (1989) of humans perpetually and seamlessly interacting with the situation they inhabit and taking their share of responsibility for that situation. Consequently, our situation is moulded by us and we are moulded by our situation. This is not a new idea. Two thousand years ago the Greek Philosopher Solon advised 'Know thy self!' (Eckroth-Bucher, 2010: 298) and in the 18th century the power of self-awareness was highly valued by the poet Robert Burns (Figure 1.3).

Table 1.1 Self-awareness exercise one

Who are you and where do you come from?
Where did you grow up?
What sort of person were you as a child? How has this changed and what things remain the same?

Talk about:

- What makes you feel happy?
- What makes you sad?
- What makes you angry?
- What makes you frustrated?
- What makes you feel passionate?

What do the answers to the questions above tell you about the sort of person you are?

List the things that have influenced you as a person:

- Your parents and other family?
- Other relationships?
- Your religion or code of life ethics?
- Entertainment personalities and media?

What do you think the flaws in those different sources of influence might be?

Table 1.2 Self-awareness exercise two

1. Talk about how someone who likes you would describe your personality.
2. Now talk about how someone who dislikes you would describe your personality.

The chances are the truth lies somewhere in between these two perspectives on you!
So having thought about the two different views of yourself, talk about the sort of person you want to be:

- Your strengths.
- Your weaknesses.
- The opportunities you have in life.
- Barriers that could prevent you getting where you want to go.
- How you might you overcome the barriers you've identified, including the help and support you might recruit.

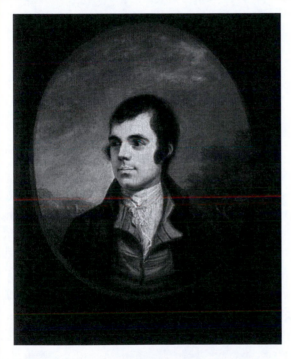

O wad some Pow'r the giftie gie us

To see oursels as others see us

It wad frae monie a blunder free us

An' foolish notion

What airs in dress an' gait wad lea'e us

An' ev'n Devotion

(Robert Burns, 1785)

This excerpt from the poem 'To a Louse' by the famous Scottish Bard goes to the heart of the goals of improved self-awareness although non Scots may require help with translation! In plain English, Burns was saying that if God would only give us the ability to see ourselves through the eyes of others we would not make so many mistakes and avoid many misguided ideas. We would change the way we dress and the things on which we spend our time. Burns' words capture the embarrassment and mental discomfort often experienced by those who are granted self-awareness through a glimpse of an audio visual recording of themselves. The poet also hints at the better world that would result if everyone was granted such an experience.

To gain insight into how we 'come across' to others we need to carefully select trusted friends or colleagues who also respect us. Other antecedents include a good memory and the ability to perceive inconsistency between our values and actions. After this we need to engage in frank, honest discussion about our strengths and weaknesses. In doing this we will have begun to achieve the self-awareness which Burns found elusive.

Figure 1.3   Robert Burns on self-awareness

Table 1.3 Self-awareness exercise three

Your social presentation (how you come across to others):

1. Describe your physical appearance:

   - Short, tall or medium height?
   - Small, large or medium frame?
   - The colour of your eyes.
   - Your hair.
   - Skin tone/colour.

2. Describe your voice:

   - Tone.
   - Usual volume.
   - Accent.

3. Think about what you do and say when you approach someone to speak to them for the first time:

   - How often do you smile?
   - Do you have a stare?
   - How do you greet them 'physically'? (Shake hands? Nod your head?)
   - What do you say to them? (Use a greeting? Just start talking?)

Now go back over numbers 1–3 and think and talk about how this appears and impacts on others. In each area think and talk about the advantages and disadvantages for you.
What can you change? What can you adjust? What effect would those changes and adjustments have on how you present to others?

A high degree of self-awareness is said to be crucial at the first encounter with any individual as a solid predictor of the level of trust and mutual respect that will characterise the ensuing relationship. We need to know how we seem to others before others can understand or benefit from us (Wilson and Crowe, 2008). This is particularly the case in emergency or acute settings where a bond of trust must be formed quickly. An example of this is given by Kirk (2007) in which a nurse in an anaesthetic room previously unknown to an anxious patient waiting to have major surgery, momentarily reassures her that she will be with her throughout the whole operation.

It is also noteworthy that being self-aware is also essential in conveying our point of view forcefully but effectively to others in times of conflict. Table 1.3 is an exercise linked to this part of the discussion. Furthermore, Wilde and Garvin (2007) argue that improved self-care is also the companion of self-awareness as self-aware people are more skilled in monitoring their own health and wellbeing.

Jack and Miller (2008) argue that there are three forms of self-awareness:

1. Cognitive. This is a conscious reasoned self-awareness: a contemporaneous understanding of body language and personal presentation or deportment; the significance of facial expression, voice and body language.

2. Affective. This is a reflective awareness; an ability to scrutinise one's perceptions and feelings together with the prejudices and assumptions these feelings may disguise. An examination of our feelings also helps us articulate nebulous situations we may otherwise struggle to describe or define.

3. Behavioural. This is reflexivity borne of self-awareness: The self-aware person is able to respond in a way that changes the world interacting with the self through a corresponding change in the self. This includes an ability to adjust one's facial expression, vocal tone and volume, body language that befits the needs of a situation.

However, real life situations call upon us to use these forms of self-awareness in combination with each other. For example, feelings can be contagious. They can begin with us but be projected onto others. Conversely, they can be at the root of other people's perspectives and generate strong feelings in us (Zembylas, 2005). Skilled self-awareness helps untangle whose emotions belong to whom in an experience and respond appropriately (Jack and Miller, 2008). Self-awareness is a prerequisite to empathy and compassion. As we explore the relationship between these notions we can begin to appreciate their importance to nursing practice.

Empathy is the ability to grasp the frame of reference of another. According to Kirk (2007: 239) to exercise empathy is:

> To understand what it is like to be in someone else's position (what it is like to live that person's life) or, perhaps less ambitious, (ii) to understand what it is like to experience phenomena as someone else experiences them.

The term 'compassion' comes from the Latin 'compati' meaning 'to suffer with'. Ballot and Campling (2011) argue that this translated meaning of the original language root is insufficient in helping us to understand the nature of compassion; the active use of empathy and kindness. Compassion moves our focus from one of self-concern to concern for others. It is defined as ' . . . sensitivity to pain and suffering in ourselves and others with a deep motivation and commitment towards alleviating and preventing it' (Gilbert and Choden, 2013: 44).

Compassion may both instigate a relationship and punctuate the course of that relationship. However, compassion and empathy require sensitivity to the feelings of another person and it is not possible to understand the feelings of another person without first understanding those feelings in ourselves. This takes self-awareness.

It is from knowledge of ourselves that we are able to articulate and understand the feelings we have experienced in different situations. From this we are able to develop empathy for others by becoming acquainted with their circumstances and imagining those circumstances to be our own. Scott (2000: 127) called this 'representational thinking' because we 'represent' the thoughts and emotions of others in our own minds. In doing so we do not need to have experienced the same type of events, but we must be able to identify and understand the feelings involved. Conversely, empathy increases self-awareness because we are increasingly mindful of our own behaviour (McQueen, 2004). Compassion and empathy are essential components in nursing (Kirk, 2007). They are tools in the skilled use of self. Compassion and empathy are needed to relate to the grief and pain of loss in family life, the sense of worthlessness and inertia of people with depression, the anxiety of parents with sick children, the displaced anger and frustration of excessive caring responsibility among relatives, to mention but a few emotional states. Without self-awareness we will experience difficulty in relating to the situations of others in a way that extends empathy to them. Moreover, we will also fail to recognise the role of our own life moulded prejudices and assumptions in the way we view others. Both will adversely affect the care we provide and how we provide it. The Johari window (Luft and Ingham, 1955) is a model of self-disclosure which has been linked to wellbeing (Figure 1.4). It has also been used to help develop greater self-knowledge.

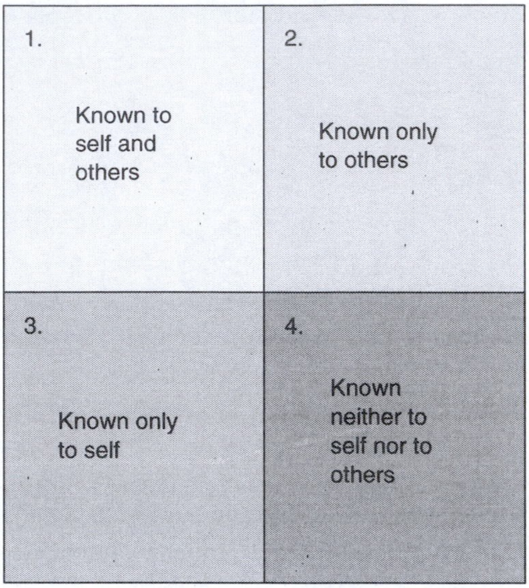

1. Known to self and others	2. Known only to others
3. Known only to self	4. Known neither to self nor to others

The Johari window was conceived by two Californian psychologists called Joe and Harry. The window is based on the philosophy that openness, self-disclosure and self-exploration in an environment of mutual trust and respect leads to greater self-knowledge, positive personal growth and development along with empowerment. The authors hold that such a process is positively related to mental health and recommend it as a simple guide for counsellors. Each window relates to a category of knowledge at work in our lives and the extent of awareness of that knowledge. The chief aim is to enlarge window number one and correspondingly reduce windows two, three and four. Activity like this in the company of trusted others is called cooperative enquiry.

Window number four contains information which is known neither to the self nor to others. This might be an undiagnosed disease with no signs or symptoms or the unrecognised abusive roots in childhood which explain some of our behaviours. **Window number three** refers to information known only to the self. This may be the memory of some thought or action from the past that haunts us and causes us needless pain or guilt. Never the less the substance of this window's content is our 'public face' or a mask we put on for the rest of the world behind which we conceal our private thoughts and insecurities. Window number three is best explored when the behaviour that constitutes our public face misrepresents us or does not serve us well. Alternatively, there will always be some matters which we wish to keep private and so some knowledge in window number three is rightly left there. **Window number two** involves information known only to others. It refers to our 'blind spot'; information so obvious in the public domain that it should be clear to us but somehow remains unknown. A crude example of this might be an individual's foul body odour or breath about which he or she is completely unaware, but of which others are only too painfully aware! In a practice situation a key worker may be unaware of how unreliable or inadequate they are for the post they hold, but colleagues choose to work around the problem this creates rather than face up to the challenge of addressing it. A family member may dominate others with whom he lives to their detriment, but be unaware of the effects of his behaviour because he has never been helped to understand them. These are examples of knowledge which is known to others but not to the self. Finally, ideally the largest window: **window number one** should contain information which is known both to others and the self. Our name is an obvious constituent here. A balanced knowledge of our strengths and weaknesses and those of others is also at home in this category. The person whose window number one is much larger than the other windows is able to live and work with others skilfully and sensitively. They are better understood and accepted for who they are.

Figure 1.4 The Johari window

Source: Luft, J. and Ingham, H. (1955) *The Johari Window: A Graphic Model for Interpersonal Relations*. University of California.

The 'self' and emotional development

Our personal background will affect our level of self-awareness and our emotional development since birth has much to offer us by way of explanation of why we think and behave as we do. This is often referred to as attachment theory. Attachment theory says that we are preprogrammed as prosocial at birth and throughout life we actively seek out the company of trusted others. This is particularly the case in times of stress and trauma when the challenges we face and the surroundings which house them are complex and unfamiliar to us, fragmenting our ability to cope and causing us to feel vulnerable. Engagement with other individuals whom we perceive as caring results in restored feelings of security, comfort and self-confidence. A failure to recruit human support results in further distress, insecurity, a lack of self-worth and even despair. This can lead to a lack of cooperation, anger, frustration and learned helplessness. Personal security (born of positive attachment patterns), on the other hand is a thinking and feeling state which promotes independence and buys time for us to regroup and plan to meet our needs. Those who have experienced positive attachment in childhood will have a balanced view of themselves and others (Belsky and Cassidy, 1994). For such people, sound self-esteem, self-confidence and self-expression together with a generous, sensitive approach to others are the order of the day. Just as someone who is financially rich has sound 'financial capital' so it can be said that someone who loves and is loved in equal measure possesses substantial 'personal capital'. Such individuals do not feel victims at the mercy of unforeseen occurrence. They are able to use their 'personal capital' to take control to meet the needs of a situation.

Theorists in psychology and mental health have long acknowledged that many people are not equipped with sound self-awareness in life (Belsky and Cassidy, 1994; Howe, Brandon, Hinnings and Schofield, 1999). An upbringing characterised by harsh criticism and lacking emotional warmth or attention can mean that a person struggles to relate to others and may not be able to gauge their contribution to a situation. Equally a child who has experienced hypersensitive care and overindulgence will sometimes struggle to relate to others as an adult. This is particularly the case where there has been perpetual conflict or where rejection has been experienced in childhood. Persons prone to anxiety arising from an emotionally abusive childhood may instinctively distrust others and hold a distorted view of others' motives.

These 'negative attachment patterns' are entirely reversible. Skilled personal investment from gifted teachers, the warmth, love, praise and encouragement from genuine friendships and partners in later life can all play a part in such a reversal. Support of this kind can result in a person with an abusive past developing self-esteem and skills which accrue personal capital. For some counseling and the support of health and social care professionals are also helpful. Consider the material in this section in conjunction with the content of Box 1.3.

Personal attachment patterns and emotionally intelligent nursing

Given that everyone who enters nursing has an emotional need met by helping others, it follows that many nurses may come from backgrounds of low warmth and high criticism. Despite many strengths and abilities these nurses may struggle to develop accurate self-awareness. For many a fear of exploring their own emotions is at the heart of this (Mazhindu, 2003). A disproportionately negative view of their faults and failings and an underestimation of their strengths will stifle a person's self-esteem and the motivation to plan innovative care. It is important to recognise this personal trait and work to address it. This begins with recognising our strengths as well as our weaknesses together with the basis for these. In doing so, rather than being unwittingly forged by our circumstances and background, we are able to choose how much we are product of them (Eckroth-Bucher, 2010). This will make it easier for us to extend the same generous measure of dealing with others, striving to achieve a view which is couched in fairness and balance rather than any satisfaction or resentment they may have generated in us.

It is clear from Jack and Miller's typology (2008) that while self-awareness, mindfulness and reflexivity are explained separately they are actually interrelated with empathy and compassion under the umbrella of emotional intelligence (Figure 1.5). Just as someone who shows themselves skillful in mathematics or verbal expression can be said to possess abstract intelligence and someone who is skilled at manipulating objects is said to have concrete intelligence, so an emotionally intelligent person has their own set of skills. Emotional intelligence is the use of self to effectively engage with and accurately interpret the emotions of others. Emotionally intelligent people are also able to organise groups and work to resolve conflict. In addition, the emotionally intelligent person is aware of their own prejudices and values together with their physical and emotional deportment regulating these as appropriate to the situation (Goleman, 1995). This latter point is the link between emotional intelligence and self-awareness.

Mindfulness

Cognitive, affective and behavioural self-awareness are closely related to a state of mindfulness (Figure 1.6). Mindfulness is a present time framed form of emotional intelligence; the application of self-awareness and empathy. It is the ability to fully resource oneself in the present moment giving attention to the needs of the 'here and now' (White, 2014). Notions of 'being present' and 'giving attention' capture a sense of being insightful as to what is meaningful and deserving of personal attention in the 'moment to moment' situation. Mindfulness operates at the exclusion of any distractions in the past, present or future. Painful or negative memories feeding present fears and prejudices which in turn might otherwise fuel anxiety over possible future scenarios are all shelved to enable one to make economic and effective use of the self. Mindfulness takes place in a setting where the mindful one is fully aware of his own thoughts, emotions and behaviours and is able to discern how these interact with those of others. Out of these considerations the mindful person is able to forge the most effective use of self.

A mindful approach in nursing is captured in the narrative by Eleanor Foster Hughes (Table 1.4). In the middle of a busy working day already punctuated with a series of challenges which stretch her coping skills, Foster Hughes is confronted by an anxious mother angry that the administration of her son's medication has been delayed. The mother and Foster Hughes bring very different perspectives to this situation. For Foster Hughes, the challenge is to focus on the needs of that moment suspending feelings of tiredness from what has already gone before and any sense of injustice that *her* needs as a human being are not being considered by others. Mindfulness also requires accepting the situation and the people in it for what they are rather than what we would like them to be. It is an informed use of self which incorporates self-awareness, an insightful knowledge of others and contemporary events. Being mindful does not mean that injustice and socially unacceptable behaviour are excused or ignored. Neither does the mindful one lack the motivation to address these issues. Instead, mindfulness is a tool of perception which supplies mental focus and prioritisation. Mindfulness ultimately produces a transformative process in Foster Hughes through more positive behaviour and in her situation through an appeased client. In this sense it is a form of reflexivity.

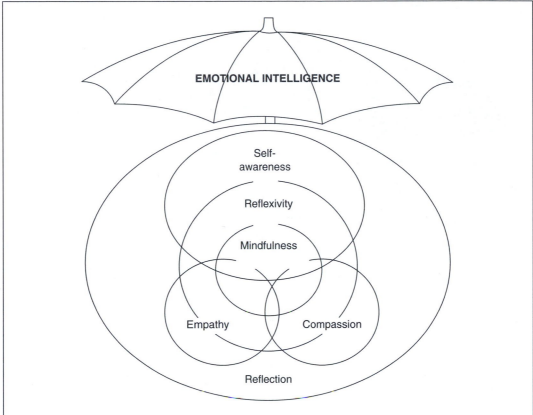

Emotional Intelligence is the use of self to move effectively in the world by optimally resourcing one's presence and personality. It is the ability to socialise with others in a positive way and shape one's behaviour on accurate interpretation of others' emotions. Self-awareness is the beginning of emotional intelligence enabling one to relate to the feelings of others through compassion and empathy. Through a conscious knowledge of one's own thoughts and feelings one is able to extend concern towards others and represent the thoughts and feelings of others in one's own mind. These qualities in turn are required to develop reflexivity and mindfulness. Mindfulness is concerned with exercising emotional intelligence 'in the present moment' deliberately excluding invasive thoughts from the past and anxieties relating to the future. Alternatively, reflexivity is able to extend emotional intelligence backwards and forwards in time to ascertain the meaning for the self, for one's life course and life meaning; 'reflexively' adapting the self in response to what is learned from a situation. While self-awareness, empathy, compassion reflexivity and mindfulness are all distinct features of emotional intelligence, they function interdependently. These facets of emotional intelligence are all facilitated by the ability to reflect on experience.

Figure 1.5   The umbrella of emotional intelligence

Reflexivity

While mindfulness is the use of self in the present moment, reflexivity is a use of self which also extends to knowledge of the past and anticipated possible futures. Reflexivity is the ability to use an experience as a 'yard stick' for the self to promote learning and positive change. As with all forms of emotional intelligence it is very much related to the idea of individuals having control over their lives.

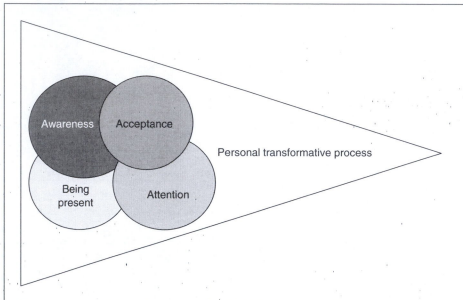

The notion of mindfulness has been defined by Kabat-Zinn (1994: 4) as 'paying attention in a particular way on purpose in the present moment and non-judgementally'. Mindfulness has five interlocking attributes:

1. Being present
2. Awareness
3. Acceptance
4. Attention which together forge a
5. Personal transformative process

Being present in a situation can lead to improved health and wellbeing through greater understanding of mind, body and emotion. 'Being present' opposes cultural approaches which value task orientation or a preoccupation with 'doing'.

Protagonists of mindfulness argue that defining a situation purely by the tasks of that situation deprives the individual of insight into its meaning. Instead mindfulness places emphasis on a way of being in the moment. Awareness is becoming deeply aware of self. It is a 'checking' or monitoring of one's feelings and understandings at the root of our behaviours and their relationship with our environment. Acceptance is the ability to accept what arises in one's awareness without resisting, avoiding or judging. Instead of reacting negatively to an experience through habitual ways of thinking, moving and doing, acceptance involves responding in a way which is crafted to suit a situation. This in turn fosters a more compassionate and forgiving attitude to the self and others, enabling us to 'accept' people and situations for what they are instead of what we would like them to be. In doing this we are able to shun destructive emotions such as anger anxiety or bitterness which squander energy better used in other ways. This builds resilience in unpleasant and challenging situations. Attention is the ability to stay in the 'moment to moment experience' without distraction from past experiences which supply unneeded anxiety, rumination and prejudice. Our coping skills are then unhindered and our responses more balance and less partial. The greater insight which accompanies self-awareness, acceptance and attention exerts a positive change or transformative process in us.

Figure 1.6   Self-awareness as part of mindfulness

Sources: Kabat-Zinn, J. (1994) *Wherever You Go There You Are: Mindfulness and Meditation in Everyday Life*. New York, Hyperion; White, L. (2014) Mindfulness in nursing: an evolutionary concept analysis. *Journal of Advanced Nursing* 70(2): 282–294.

Table 1.4 Being mindful
By Eleanor Foster-Hughes, RSCN

Being present
Amid a chaotic clinical setting with implications for the future as well as the present, Eleanor Foster Hughes remains 'in the moment'. She is ready and willing to be with an anxious mother despite the fact that James' needs may rightly have taken second place behind other priorities. She absorbs the full thrust of Cara's presence and attitude. This helps Foster Hughes to sharpen her attention and awareness.

Attention
Eleanor is not distracted by other immediate or pending pressures. This enables her to remain focused on Cara's presentation and the importance of shaping her own impact on this. This sense of focus helps the nurse to suspend any distaste for Cara's hostility and keep shelved underlying concerns about herself or her family. This leaves Foster Hughes free to address the present situation effectively with self-awareness,

It's 5.15pm and it has not been a good day. Social services and the police have just left following a formal safeguarding children investigation that has taken all my time so far today. Two nurses scheduled for the night shift ahead have just phoned in sick. I have not even tried to get cover yet because we are busy comforting the parents of a 4-year-old girl who has just gone down to the operating suite.

In the wake of all of this Cara is facing me down telling me that her son James was due his medication 5 minutes ago. James has been a patient on our floor for several weeks and his mother has been a permanent feature on the landscape for most of this time. Cara is not an educated woman but she has an acid tongue and she's armed with a brand of sardonic sarcasm that makes me wonder if someone in the media writes her scripts for her. She has had some of the junior staff in tears before now and you could be forgiven for thinking she enjoys it.

I must stay focused. It won't help to think about how tired I am or that I haven't had a break since I came on duty. It won't help to think about my mother whose biopsy result is due the day after tomorrow. The telephone is ringing but someone else can answer it. Someone is calling my name but they can wait. I take a long, quiet, slow, deep breath. Like so many parents in her position Cara knows her son's condition and care plan as well if not better than many of the practitioners looking after him. This makes her powerful and intimidating to anyone who pretends to know more than they actually do and is reluctant to share decision making with her. I must always show that I am listening to her and acting on what she is saying.

(continued)

Table 1.4 *(continued)*

Awareness

Foster Hughes is aware of the prejudices and assumptions her own presentation can engender in Cara. She is able to exercise empathy for Cara's situation and life story. Self-awareness and empathy act together to inform the nurse's response; lowering her height by sitting down and speaking softly as she acknowledges Cara's concerns to deescalate tension.

Telling the story

Eleanor forestalls the negative effect any frustration she might have experienced over Cara's lack of appreciation for nursing effort accepting her patient's mother for who and what she is. She also 'accepts' that a successful outcome will be measured in the context of Cara's anger and fear relating to her son and the tragic events that have featured heavily in her life. Nevertheless Cara's response shows that the nurse's mindfulness and empathy have reaped a reward.

I put myself in her shoes for an instant, how would I feel living my life in front of everybody else knowing that no matter what we do for her son, nothing seems to be working? She has so many questions and we have no answers. None. I'm standing there in my pristine blue uniform, a figure in authority who is supposed to be an expert. I am taller and slimmer than Cara. I know my clipped voice and old fashioned 'English actress' accent irritate her and give her the impression I look down on her. She has expected so much of me but it seems I can deliver nothing for this woman. Cara's hostility and sarcasm are borne of her frustration, anger and fear. This is no secret. She lost her husband in Afghanistan and now she is afraid she is going to lose her son. She is not going to change. Even if James recovers it is unlikely that Cara will give the nursing team the credit that we will deserve. But James is still my patient and his needs and those of his mother's are as great as those of a family who thank you every time you do something for them and buy you half a sweet shop when they are discharged.

I sit down on a spare play stool close to where Cara is standing. Cara is now looking down at *me*. I lower my voice to a stage whisper.

'I'm really sorry Cara. I'm going to get his drugs ready right away.'

I get up, turn around and walk back towards the nurses' station.

'I won't hold my breath!' replies Cara.

She appears defiant but there is a difference. Her voice is lower and more subdued than before. I have appeased her although this will never be acknowledged out loud. I don't reply but keep walking. I know she is still frustrated, angry and afraid.

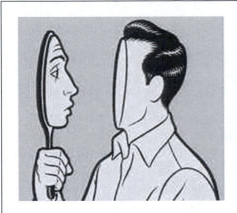

Alan Peshkin's theory seeks to promote improved self-awareness through exploration of one's experiences and the emotions they arouse. Peshkin (1988: 1) argued that subjectivity was like a 'garment that cannot be removed'. He believed it was foolish to purport objectivity and that it made sense to clarify the role of one's motives and preference in the course of his research rather than declaring them at the end. Peshkin uncovered in himself six subjective 'I's identified in the course of his work. He describes how his values and interests steered him to linger in enquiry in some areas but not in others. For example his interest in those who sought to preserve their ethnic identity led to his discovery of his ethnic maintenance 'I', and the deep sense of empathy felt for parents who felt their community was unjustly denigrated by inhabitants of surrounding towns led to his discovery of his justice seeking 'I'.

Peshkin's approach to narrative, examining what holds our interest and provokes core emotions in us, provides the reflective practitioner with portals through which to view themselves. It also provides the reader with a glimpse as to where and when the subject and subjective self became joined together with the impact they had on each other. This approach was captured in a nursing culture by Bradbury-Jones et al. (2009) in their approach to student nurse journaling. Bradbury-Jones and her team were able to show increased self-awareness among students through their application of Peshkin's approach. There is an opportunity to try out Peshkin's ideas in the exercise in Table 1.1.

Figure 1.7   Peshkin's theory on improved self-awareness: the subjective 'I'

A reflexive person repeatedly uses experience as a learning tool to redesign their lives. Any situation can be used positively as a tool to teach us more about who we are. Alan Peshkin's theory (Figure 1.7) is built on this assumption. Peshkin developed a method of self-awareness by exploring the emotions he experienced in different settings. The exercise in Table 1.1 provides an opportunity to try out Peshkin's method.

To the reflexive person life choices, personality traits, family, education and work are all seen as mouldable. Reflexive people ask questions such as 'What does this have to do with me?', 'What does this say about the sort of person I am?' and 'How does this experience fit into my life or give my life meaning; where I am, the sort of person I want to be and where I want to go?' We should also remember that reflexive exercises may well bring to mind positive personality strengths which can be developed further.

Box 1.2 contains a short excerpt from a long reflective narrative by Emma Oram, a nursing student in her first year of study at the time of writing. Emma became intrigued with a woman in her care suffering with a personality disorder who insisted on carrying a bag of fresh food with her everywhere she went. Time spent in conversation with the woman and further enquiry into her case revealed the explanation for the woman's behaviour. The woman had suffered abuse from an early age and mental disorder from young adulthood. Her three children were removed from her at birth and placed in alternative care by social services. She never saw them again. Carrying a bag of food meant that the woman would be able to feed her children if ever they came back and found her again.

Box 1.2   Reflexivity and biographicity: food for thought

By Emma Oram

This situation helped me reframe my life as a whole in terms of how fortunate I am. It made me think about how unpredictable life is. This woman's condition was life changing from the time she gave birth. She was once, a beautiful young girl with dreams, hopes of happiness like everyone else . . . never in a million years could she have imagined herself living in a rehabilitation ward, with an illness that she could not control, on medication for the rest of her life with independence lost forever. Nor could anyone have predicted such circumstances. In this moment I realised that my vocation is to help this woman and many others like her suffering from mental health disorders. I woke up to the real need present among those who suffer severe mental illness. My involvement with this woman has made me resolve to set goals for my future career as a registered mental health nurse; to become skilled in active listening and therapeutic counselling; equipped with empathy and compassion; to be an advocate for the disadvantaged and the vulnerable in our society and promote their empowerment and wellbeing.

The impact of this patient's tragic life story on Oram is an example of reflexivity. Oram is helped to 'reframe her life' in the face of the unfortunate situation of another. 'Reframing' means to take a different perspective on a situation in the light of other evidence about which one has been previously unaware. By reframing Oram is able to realise how fortunate she is in her life when compared with the plight of someone who suffers from a severe mental illness. Moreover, the lack of natural justice in her patient's life history, the unpredictable nature of the woman's life course when set against her strengths and opportunities in youth impacts on Oram's own philosophy on life. She is able to articulate clearly her rationale for nursing study and her goals beyond graduation. These may have been known to her before but the experience of caring for someone who is severely mentally ill has added greater meaning to this. For Oram her reflexive thought is the start of a journey towards professional maturity. Oram chooses her role and exercises influence on her life course interacting positively with her experience rather than being a passive recipient of time and unforeseen circumstance. This method of using an experience to reshape one's life course and life meaning in a fulfilling way is called biographicity (Illeris, 2007).

Reflexivity provides the opportunity to use a situation to examine ourselves. An immature response to a situation is to see it purely in terms of the actions of others as if we were passive observers of every experience. Feelings of fear and embarrassment, joy and satisfaction, anxiety and anger, sadness and frustration arising from an experience can be explored and used to inform us about ourselves.

Self-awareness, mindfulness and reflexivity all resource compassion and empathy and are related to each other as forms of emotional intelligence.

Conclusion

Some professions largely depend on the skilled use of physical or biochemical knowledge. However, because of the importance of the nurse–patient relationship in the provision of care, optimum practice in nursing depends first on self-awareness; the effective use of self. Moreover, good reflective practice rests on balanced knowledge of the self and one's impact on others. Self-awareness is

Box 1.3 About yourself

Reading a chapter like this may well have caused you to begin to think about yourself in more depth; your upbringing, your personality, your fears, hopes, strengths and weaknesses. This is entirely positive. If any of this causes you distress you must not regret having started out on what is an important journey of discovery. Get help and support wherever you can. Talk to trusted friends, personal tutors, or your family doctor about what is troubling you. Most colleges and centres of higher education provide a free confidential counselling service. These services exist because you are not the only learner to find increased self-awareness initially painful. Take courage from knowing that this also means that you have the power to change for the better.

Exploring the detail of reflecting on one's experience begins in Chapter 2 but you may find it helpful to begin writing about yourself and your feelings now. There is no magic formula for doing this well. Just start writing. Expressing yourself on paper will also stimulate you to think more as you become your own listener. Standish, Smeyers and Smith (2010) describe how someone in the role of reader often becomes aware of aspects of what is written about which the writer is not aware. This helps us to understand why writing and then reading what one has written can prove to be a reflective exercise in itself. By beginning a private journal of this kind you may become more relaxed about exploring your personality and its roots. If certain passages and phrases prove useful for future written work then this is all for the better. These are important skills in becoming a reflective practitioner.

conscious knowledge of how one presents to others together with our underpinning motives and values. Self-awareness is possible because we are sentient beings conscious of our place in space and time. Self-awareness arising out of a balanced view of one's own strengths and weaknesses together with our own social presentation is essential in establishing relationships of trust with others. Self-aware people also take better care of themselves. The quality of our self-awareness will depend on the quality of positive emotional attachments in our own lives. Self-awareness is also the basis for the representational thinking on which compassion and empathy can be experienced. Exercises in self-discovery are conducive to improved self-awareness and mental wellbeing. The use of self involves the sensitive and skillful use of one's personality and presence to achieve positive outcomes in relationships. Reflexivity is the ability to use a situation as a yardstick for the self and the tailoring of a response that is moulded by one's experience of that situation. Reflexivity is the use of situations to examine ourselves with a view to self-improvement. Reflexivity is closely related to biographicity: the reshaping of one's life meaning and life course through use of experience. Mindfulness is the informed use of self in the present moment deploying a present time related form of reflexivity.

Time should be taken to absorb the import of this chapter before moving on to other sections of the book. It should be clear that a skill such as reflection which is integral to the use of self rests on accurate and uncensored knowledge of the self and a willingness to address deficits. Much self-deception and pointless time consuming storytelling which results in no genuine learning about the self or one's practice can be avoided through the preliminary self-examination encouraged in this section.

The failure of many nurses to fully benefit from reflective practice does not lie with reflection as a method of learning but in a lack of heed and respect paid to development of the necessary personal qualities and other prerequisites which are discussed in Chapter 2.

2 Becoming a reflective practitioner – part two

Exploring the art of reflection

Box 2.1   Main points: Chapter 2

- Reflection is a way of thinking about our experiences to give them meaning.
- The process of reflection will only be enabled when all the necessary personal and environmental prerequisites are in place.
- Reflection for professional practice works best when both internal and external evidence are considered.
- Sharing our reflections helps us appreciate the value of stories to learning.
- Reflective practice can help nurses demonstrate accountability and self-regulation.
- Reflective practice helps prevent complacency and habitualisation.

Introduction

Chapter 1 was concerned with the importance of self-awareness and the understanding of the use of self as a personal 'starter pack' for engaging in reflection. In contrast this chapter will discuss the remaining essential qualities in the course of defining and explaining the process. Storytelling and personal biography are age old methods of preserving and challenging values across cultures and generations. This notion will be used to highlight the learning potential of reflective narrative and a definitive line will be drawn between this and that of an academic essay with which reflection is often confused. A few words of caution will also be offered. The deeply personal and fragile nature of reflection will be stressed together with the implications this has for teaching and learning. Consideration will also be given to ethical issues arising from reflective practice.

Turning experience into learning

Experience is of itself worthless unless it has meaning for us. When our experience has meaning it can inform how we behave in the future (Friere, 1971). This should help us to see why merely having been a parent does not necessarily imply knowledge about good child care or good child rearing. Neither does it imply that someone who has 20 years of nursing experience is necessarily a good nurse.

Parents become good parents by learning from their mistakes and building on their successes. They think back over situations which may have gone well or which may not have gone as they planned or hoped. Good parents listen and consider the views and feelings of their children; not just their own. They are aware of their own personal strengths and weaknesses. Good parents consult expert guidance in books, on television and on the internet along with advice from other parents whose judgement they respect. This new knowledge is then applied to future parenting with due thought being given to changing circumstances. Good parents also share the learning from their experiences with others. This way of thinking on our interpretation of experience to give it meaning; drawing on internal and external sources of knowledge turns experience into learning. It is called reflection (Boud, Keogh and Walker, 1985).

Reflection is a way of thinking about an experience retrospectively, considering and reconsidering the sights, sounds, smells, tastes and even tactile stimuli of a situation together with the thoughts and emotions they generated in us and may have generated in others who were involved.

Defining reflection in nursing practice

Reflection is a highly personal and individual activity so we should not be surprised that there are many definitions which are at variance with one another. However, reflection as it forms part of professional practice has been described by Wilkinson (1999: 36). She says:

> Reflective practice is an *active process* whereby the professional can gain an *understanding of how historical, social, cultural, cognitive and personal experiences have contributed to professional knowledge* acquisition and practice. An examination of such factors yields an opportunity to identify new potentials within practice, thus *challenging the constraints of habituated thoughts and practices.*

So reflection is an active process. We choose to do it. Self-discipline is required to lend focus and direction. It is therefore not the same as daydreaming. It is not about copying what others do. Nor is it simply evaluation. Evaluation is the judgment of the value of an experience in which the original goals or what we set out to do are compared with outcomes; what we actually end up with. True reflection is about examining all the layers of an experience and identifying pointers for learning (Hannigan, 2001).

Reflective practice in nursing is the application of the principles of reflection to nursing practice. Good nurses like good parents think deeply on situations which are exemplars for good practice but also on negative experiences. Good nurses consider the views and feelings of their colleagues and of patients and patients' families not just their own. Good nurses are mature individuals who know their strengths and weaknesses and take these into account in a realistic reflection on any situation. Reflective nurses will access the knowledge of more experienced colleagues as an apprentice learns from a master worker. However, they will not do this with blind faith in 'copycat' fashion but in conjunction with other sources of expertise. This means searching formal databases containing peer reviewed journals of research and theory, expert guidance from specialist organisations, social

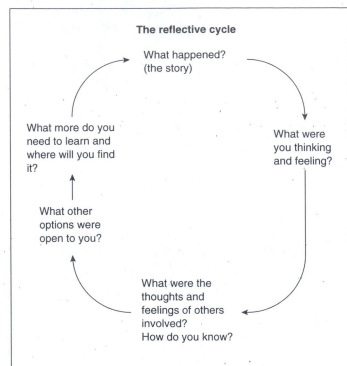

The reflective cycle

What happened?
(the story)

What were
you thinking
and feeling?

What were the
thoughts and
feelings of others
involved?
How do you know?

What other
options were
open to you?

What more do you
need to learn and
where will you find
it?

For a beginner, reflection is best understood as a cyclical activity in which one part of the process leads on to another. The model illustrated here is loosely based on Gibbs (1988). After choosing an experience you should begin by telling the story or remembering exactly what happened. Research into truth telling (Johnson and Raye 1998) has shown that one is unlikely to remember all the facts in chronological order and may have to return to certain points to fill in some details or amend realised errors. Research cycling; processing the experience or a specific part of it through the reflective cycle again is very useful. In fact, the more one does this the more is likely to be learned (Boud et al. 1985). The police use this method to great effect in their interviews with both witnesses and suspects to establish as clear a picture of an event as possible (Vrij 2000).

After this describe your feelings and thoughts at the time of the experience. Research in neural science (Damassio 2000) has shown that we all feel before we think and that our emotions often open the gate to information which has been hidden from conscious thought. Immordino-Yang and Damassio (2007) have shown how emotion acts like a 'rudder' to guide our thinking so reflecting on our emotions is always useful. Depending on the experience, we may find ourselves reliving the emotions generated all over again. Provided that we remain relatively composed, this will actively help the reflective process. Try to establish the reasoning behind your actions. Next, try to contemplate what the thoughts, values, beliefs and feelings of others involved in the situation might have been. After this, it is important to ask what led you to these conclusions. Among the features that might be considered are body language, facial expression and vocal tone. This will help uncover and confront any assumptions, prejudices or value judgements which we may have been harboured. This is internal evidence. Following this, try to consider other options that might have been available and therefore other courses that might have been taken. Finally try to establish what external evidence exists to support or refute your conclusions. This will involve gathering academically credible evidence such as peer reviewed journal papers from a data base search, expert guidance from specialist organisations, government policy documents or professional codes of practice. Remember this knowledge is personal to you. So without sharing this with others either through discussion or writing, no one will ever know and the knowledge will be lost. This is why the final phase of making recommendations for your future practice is important. In this way reflection is a way of helping you to understand yourself and helping others to understand you. On completion of the reflective cycle you should know:

1. What knowledge and principles are transferrable to future contexts?
2. What evidence is there to support this?
3. How does this inform my nursing practice?

Figure 2.1 The cycle of reflection

policy and professional codes of ethics which are relevant to the experience. This is external evidence. Figure 2.1 provides basic guidance on engaging with the reflective process.

In education, learning outcomes or competencies are often used to demonstrate learning achievement. Yet these are, by themselves, crude measures of learning because they do not show *how* the student learns; the methods that worked for them and those that left them confused, the chance detours and corrected misunderstandings along the way. On the other hand, reflection explains how the learning outcome was reached and how we become competent in the tasks of practice. After this the nurse can move forward better informed about her practice having carefully reflected on experience in the light of research, theory and other guidance. The nurse with twenty year's experience subjected to reflection is not like the nurse 'set in her ways' whose practice and practice planning are habituated. The nurse who is a reflective practitioner draws on a meaningful body of knowledge grounded in life long learning. She does not 'rest on her laurels' but continues to use reflection to turn her experience into learning.

Reflective writing is different from academic writing. It is true that reflection can be used within an academic piece of work but they are not the same. Writing an essay on a given subject requires nothing more than a grasp of the literature on that subject and a good writing style. Reflective writing requires more. Reflective writing is first more personal and second draws on a wider range of knowledge than an academic essay to help learning (Boud, 2010). Reflection tells us about the 'knowing from the living', the 'knowing in the doing' and the 'knowing from the doing' (Polanyi, 1999; Billet, Smith and Barker, 2005).

The knowing from the living

A man can write a book about how to be a good husband. He may discuss a wide range of subjects relating to building and maintaining a good relationship: communication skills, understanding and empathising with women, forgiveness, being a good sexual partner, teamwork and division of roles in a relationship, managing decisions such as if and when to have children. The author may attempt to add credibility to his arguments by referencing and weaving research findings in psychology into his text. Still at the end of the book the reader does not even know if the author is or ever has been married. We are given no practical glimpse of how his advice is applied. Worse still, if it transpires that the man is married and his wife considers him a poor partner his book is discredited. Alternatively, suppose the man writes about his own experiences of marriage, sharing his successes and openly discussing his mistakes weaved into his arguments. He then compares and contrasts his experiences with relevant research. This is a much more powerful piece of work. His honest personal account of his lived experience of marriage wins respect from the reader and we are all able to learn from his experience inclusive of his mistakes and successes. This is the knowing from the living.

The knowing in the doing

The skills we use in life all rest on a reliable knowledge base but they also validate that knowledge base. In other words, the theoretical knowledge is of little value without the ability to apply it. For example, cooking an omelette or riding a bicycle are both skills gained on the back of scientific knowledge, but reading a book about either is of little value to someone who has not attempted to cook or never rode a bicycle. A text on the process of cooking an omelette; the importance of fresh eggs kept at room temperature, the optimum heat level for the pan and the correct amount of oil and the consistency of the omelette which signals that they are ready to serve is only helpful when the reader attempts to put the knowledge into action. Only when the reader attempts to cook an omelette for the first time does he appreciate the skill in bringing the actions together in a polished performance. In the same way a book about how to ride a bike may discuss the importance of adjusting the height of the saddle, pushing off effectively, achieving forward movement through pedalling and looking straight ahead to maintain balance, but the reader does not *learn* how to ride a bicycle by reading a book but by *actively riding it*. By actively getting on a bicycle and applying the theory she knows, she is able to overcome her fears, endure repeatedly falling off, understand the gain of forward momentum which in turn helps her achieve balance and fuel her confidence. This polished performance is competence. It is testimony to embodied knowing. Our bodies' have the ability to carry out our wishes with precision and also inform our minds through sensory messages. Embodied knowledge is knowledge in a behavioural context; knowing in the doing (Laurence, 2012). Such competence in body and mind is achieved with practise and nearly always more speedily achieved with the encouragement of a teaching expert; interaction between 'master worker' and 'apprentice' (Polanyi, 1998).

Reflection captures the knowing in the doing. Good narratives are punctuated with accounts of how apprehensive or excited the learner may have been prior to the new experience. Narratives give systematic accounts of learning in action: honest declarations of ignorance of some elements of the skill being learned, misunderstandings of the underlying theory and how they were clarified culminating in the sweet feeling of sheer joy and pride when competence is achieved. Reflective narratives frequently feature expressions such as 'I never realised', 'Now I understand' or 'It was then that it suddenly occurred to me'. So reflection helps us see beyond the competence tick boxes and learning outcomes to reveal the knowing in the doing. Notice for example Stephanie Forrest's account of her interaction with a depressed patient (Table 2.1). As Stephanie's story unfolds we are helped to see how she confirms for herself the combined value of stimulating recreation, personal support and drug treatment. In doing so she is able to realise a new level of confidence and self-worth.

The knowing from the doing

When my father attempted to teach me how to ride a bicycle his lack of sensitivity and teaching skill were all too apparent. He placed me on a bicycle at the brow of a hill with his hand on the back of the saddle. After telling me to pedal forward he let go his hand from the back of the bicycle and cried 'Okay! You're on your own!'. Several skinned elbows, shins and knees later, competence still proved elusive to me. I later learned that as a young boy my father learned to ride a bicycle in this same fashion at the hands of some older boys in his neighbourhood. The fact that by some miracle he stayed on the bicycle on the first attempt had been enough to convince him that this same method would suffice for me. Most crucially it was enough to convince me that more effort, encouragement and empathy would be required when I taught my own son.

Bruner (1999: 114) advises that a good teacher must 'know what it is like not to know'. In the course of practice life we encounter many good teachers who inspire us along with some professed teachers who are best forgotten. On being enabled to develop a skill well we often recall the previous occasions we were taught the same skill poorly and wonder why those other practice teachers

Table 2.1 The games people play
By Stephanie Forrest, first year nursing student

Telling the story
A piece of reflection should always begin with the story. By doing this you set the context for yourself and anyone who reads the narrative or listens to what you have to say. Tell the truth as you perceive and recall it. Telling the story will help bring more detail back to your mind. This will mean that you have to return to different parts of the text to insert this detail into the story to keep the account in chronological order.

Feelings
Always reserve space to describe your feelings at the time and try to ascertain the feelings of others from the evidence available in the experience. Notice how this helps Stephanie to realise her progress as an effective member of the nursing team. In addition she is also able to ascertain her practice teacher's positive feelings from the behavioural evidence at hand.

Tony had been really withdrawn and quite monosyllabic despite all sorts of attempts to engage with him. I would try to talk to him but never felt I had the skill or experience. Then I noticed the table tennis table was free. It's amazing how knocking that ball back and forward across a tiny net suddenly brought him out of himself. He started to talk about his mother and her gambling addiction. It turns out that Tony blamed himself as a child for this and to a large extent still does. It was as if playing a game together broke the ice between us and helped Tony to relax. It only occurred to me after that he must have trusted me. I've known for some time that patients with depression or psychotic illness have problems concentrating and I know that playing chess or table tennis can help this but today I saw this work right in front of me. No one on the team knew about Tony's mum until I told them. My practice teacher looked surprised and then quickly thanked me.

 I felt a powerful surge of self-worth and confidence. It was as if suddenly I was a nurse who made a difference instead of an observer who didn't have much of a clue. I could see my practice teacher was pleased that my interaction with a patient was proving productive.

(continued)

Table 2.1 *(continued)*

The external evidence
Notice that in considering a piece of external evidence to further inform her reflection, Stephanie changes from the first person ('I') to the third person when describing the findings of others. This is an important habit to develop as it will help you to think abstractly about the transferrable principles at work in your story.

NMC competencies
It is good practice to index the pertinent NMC competences if you are using the narrative as additional evidence of your learning. Nurses working outside the UK should use the learning indices of their own regulatory body.

References
Always reference any external evidence which you use to inform your narrative.

Begley (2005) states that medication is often more effective when combined with nursing strategies such as this. Games and other pastimes aimed at prolonging concentration and stimulating self-esteem can impact positively on a person's mood faster than it takes an antidepressant to be absorbed, distributed, metabolised and reach therapeutic plasma levels. So two things happened here today. I saw theory meld with practice because by helping Tony to trust me and talk about himself. And by acting on it, I also became a valued member of the team.

NMC Competencies
1.3; 1.7; 1.9; 2.1; 2.2.; 2.3; 2.4; 2.6; 3.7; 4.2.

Reference
Begley, J. (2005) Bridging the concentration gap with depressed patients: nursing strategies. *The British Journal of Mental Health Nursing.* 42(6): 24–29

could not have explained matters so fully, so simply and so well. We may also consider that our confidence would have grown more rapidly had we been treated with more empathy and kindness. This reflection helps us realise a better way of learning from a poor way of teaching. We have learned *how not* to teach others. Our memories of our injured feelings help us infuse empathy and compassion into teaching our own students. It is a way of using negative experiences to inspire better practice in ourselves and others. This is the knowing from the doing. However, there is another way in which reflection informs our practice.

Reflection on experience should start us on a road of discovery learning. The reflective practitioner may then add academic credibility by supporting, comparing and contrasting his experience with expert guidance and research evidence. This is the third difference between reflective narrative and an essay: a good essay will show someone's research and theoretical knowledge informing and challenging the way we behave in practice. A good reflective narrative will inform and challenge the way we behave in practice but it may also contain messages from experience of practice to challenge and inform established theory. Miller's competency pyramid (1990) (Figure 2.2)

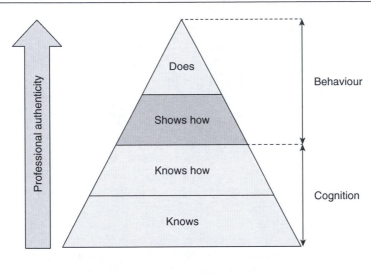

Miller's competency pyramid illustrates how a learner progresses towards professional authenticity or competency through four stages of personal knowledge. The base level (Knows) is one of factual knowledge. The learner is able to hold a detailed discussion around the body of knowledge relevant to a particular practice skill. At the second level the learner is able to discuss how the factual knowledge can be applied in practice (Knows how). At the third level (Shows how) the learner is able to behaviourally demonstrate the application of the factual knowledge in practice. Finally competency is achieved when the learner is able to integrate the evidence based practice skill within everyday behaviour. 'Knowing' and 'Knowing how' represent the cognitive dimension of skill. 'Showing how' and 'Doing' represent cognition in a behavioural context. Different forms of assessment are appropriate for different layers of the pyramid. For example direct observation should be used for 'Doing' and OSCE's can be used for 'Showing how'. Essays, tests and Questionnaires can be used for 'Knows' and 'Knows how'. However, only reflective narratives can bring together knowledge from all four layers retrospectively by integrating theory with the knowing from the living, the knowing in the doing and the living from the doing.

Figure 2.2   Miller's competency pyramid

Source: Miller, G. E. (1990) The Assessment of Clinical Skills/Competence/Performance. *Academic Medicine* 65(9): 563–567.

demonstrates how the progression from textbook knowing to competence in practice takes place and how this can be captured in a narrative. Wilson and Crowe (2008) also described the formal and informal knowledge combination used by practitioners to forge optimum practice. Questions are produced from reflection on your experience which inform, challenge and demand refinement of theory and policy requiring further research into the issues that have been identified. This is called closing the theory practice gap. Note how both Stephanie Forrest (Table 2.1) and Marie Girdham (Table 2.2) weave current theoretical knowledge into their reflections to bolster their learning. However, their experiences also confirm the rectitude of the referenced sources they cite.

Fostering effective reflection

There are a number of personal qualities, abilities and conditions that must be in place for effective reflection to take place. Figure 2.3 shows why the balance between these factors is essential to reflection through application of Illeris' tension triangle. Personal qualities, abilities and a positive learning environment all matter and are inter-related. Two of the personal qualities; self-awareness and reflexivity were discussed in Chapter 1.

Table 2.2 Leg ulcers
By Marie Girdham, first year nursing student

The descriptive or 'story' part of a reflective piece can vary in size. If the story is long it is wise to confine it to an appendix. In Marie's case it is very brief. Once again notice the role of her feelings, in that discomfort over her lack of pathological knowledge is what moves her to want to learn more. Reflection on Maclaren (2002) provides her with the professional justification for this.

In the course of my first community placement I became aware of the prevalence of people suffering with leg ulcers. It seemed every other patient had some sort of leg ulcer of varying size shape and smell. I wondered why they were so prevalent, and what caused them in the first place. Realising that I knew little about the pathology of this condition despite having learned about their nursing care, left me feeling uncomfortable. *Maclaren (2002) explains how continuing professional education is the bridge between nurses as thinkers and knowers and nurses as merely doers. It follows from this that I need to understand the evidence underpinning the care I provide.*

A leg ulcer is a chronic break in the layer of cells that form the surface of the skin in the lower leg excluding forefoot or toes (Simon, Dix and McCollum, 2004). This is the stage at which most patients seek treatment and this is why the management of leg ulcers by promoting epithelialisation is a major part of modern community nursing. The ulcer is secondary to problems associated with reduced oxygenation within the limb's circulatory circuit which lead to localised deterioration of tissue including the skin.

The blood vessels serving the lower limb are most notably the Long and Short Saphenous veins, and perforating veins that connect the two. The associated arteries are the Femoral Artery and the Popliteal Artery which is a continuation of the Femoral Artery, and runs posterior, anterior and centrally to the tibia (Tortora and Derrickson, 2006). Venous leg ulcers are associated with venous insufficiency and valvular incompetence within the Saphenous Veins and are the more common type of leg ulceration (Negus, 2005). District nurses have been shown to spend up to half their time treating this condition (Simon et al., 2004) which explains the prevalence of leg ulcer care and clinics which I witnessed in my placement! In health, leg muscles contract aiding the transport of blood flow against the gravitational force placed on it.

Marie's discussion of leg ulcers could easily have been in more depth particularly pertaining to the aetiology of the condition, but remember this is a personal statement of learning, not an academic essay. What is important is that the new learning is related back to her own experience. Notice her correlation of Simon et al.'s findings (2004) with her own observations on placement.

Valves formed by extraversions of the endothelium and tunica media with muscular bundles connected at their base open and close to seal the progress of circulation and prevent backlog or reflux.

However, in the presence of vascular or valve disease, reflux occurs causing venous hypertension, oedema, pigmentation, swelling, heaviness and pain. An additional clinical sign is brown staining called lipodermatosclerosis. This is a brown staining resulting from the impact of backlog on less muscular capillaries leading to leakage (Negus, 2005). The role of the leg muscles in the circulation of blood in the lower limbs shows the essential part played by mobility and weight control in the promotion of effective venous drainage. Good nutrition also plays a part (Simon et al., 2004).

In contrast to a venous leg ulcer, an arterial leg ulcer is caused by reduction of arterial blood supply often caused by atherosclerotic plaque which narrows the lumen. The result is hypoxaemia and necrosis. A less frequent cause is the formation of thrombo embolism (Kumar, Cotran and Robbins, 2003).

In the final section, Marie returns to 'life' to apply what she has learned; breathing greater meaning into her grasp of her grandfather's disease experience and providing her practice with a deeper knowledge which helps her see beyond the task of wound care to issues of prevention and patient partnership.

An improved understanding of the patho-physiology of leg ulcers has personal and professional meaning for me. It has personal meaning because my grandfather was diagnosed with a venous leg ulcer secondary to venous thrombosis 4 years ago. Following a severe onset of arthritis my grandfather had resorted to excessive rest. The first clinical signs he showed were pain and unilateral swelling in one ankle and then an ulcer. I still remember being perplexed by the level of pain and discomfort he suffered. The ulcer healed with a combination of wound treatments and compression bandaging. Interestingly he was encouraged to increase his physical exercise and now, in good health, helps prevent the return of the ulcer by taking regular long walks. His experience helps me bring to my studies of the condition to life. Understanding leg ulcers has professional meaning for me

(continued)

Table 2.2 *(continued)*

because awareness of the underlying causes means that I no longer view the condition as another wound which needs to be dressed. There are underlying causes which can be prevented by working in partnership with the patient to promote mobility commensurate with the patient's health status, improve nutrition and attempt weight control. In this way the patient can be empowered to take charge of their own recovery.

References

Kumar, V, Cotran, RS, and Robbins, SI. (2003) *Basic Pathology* (7th Edition). Philadephia. Saunders.

Maclaren, J. (2002) Reflecting on your expert practice. *Nursing Times* 98(9): 38–39

Negus, D, (2005) *Leg Ulcers: Diagnosis and Management* (Third Edition). Oxford. Taylor and Francis.

Simon, DA, Dix, FP, McCollum, CN. (2004) The Management of Venous Leg Ulcers. *British Medical Journal*, 328(7452): 1358–1362.

Tortora, G, Derrickson, B. (2006) *Principles of Anatomy and Physiology.* Hoboken, New Jersey. John Wiley and Sons Ltd.

Marie is sure to list her sources of supportive evidence in the references.

Honest and creativity

Make a contract with yourself to *be honest*. The need to preserve credibility and self-esteem by self-justification is strong in everyone (Mezirow, 1981). However, students who fabricate their reflective accounts, seek to justify or elevate themselves through adjusted versions of events or tell their lecturer or practice teacher what they think they want to hear, waste their time and learn nothing. Be yourself and be creative in your writing. Accept that this is your perspective on what happened and that there may be other points of view (Bradbury-Jones, Hughes, Murphy, Parry and Sutton, 2009).

Time, space, peace and quiet

Give respect to time, space and privacy. It is no surprise that all great philosophers have been lovers of solitary walking and that conversely many of us in our busy, hurried age are robbed of precious reflection time. This is not least because we are so accessible and distracted through technology such as social networking, email, mobile phones, tablets and pagers. Amid such communication chaos,

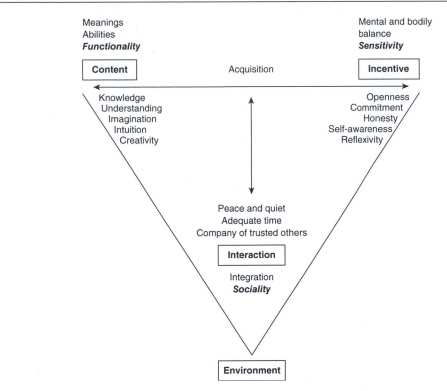

Meanings
Abilities
Functionality

Content   Acquisition   **Incentive**

Mental and bodily
balance
Sensitivity

Knowledge
Understanding
Imagination
Intuition
Creativity

Openness
Commitment
Honesty
Self-awareness
Reflexivity

Peace and quiet
Adequate time
Company of trusted others

Interaction

Integration
Sociality

Environment

Knud Illeris (2007) argued that learning can be represented within a 'tension triangle' with three dimensions and two processes. The three dimensions are the content, the incentive and the environment. **The content** comprises of what the person already knows and the skills such as understanding and imagination which they use to develop their knowledge base by discerning meaning in experience that supplies learning opportunities. Content is what permits the individual to function as a learner. **The incentive** comprises of those qualities which permit development of sensitivity to the environment in which we seek to learn. These would include humility, openness, honesty and self-awareness. These are the ingredients required to rebalance the disequilibrium which is the conscious state of not knowing. **The environment** is the social setting in the context of the society and culture in which the learner lives and interacts. **The content** and **the incentive** make up **the acquisition process**. The environment interacting with the individual forms **the interactive process**. The interactive process recognises that no one truly learns alone. It facilitates sociality in the learner as he immerses himself in new experiences and integrates them within a social context. The triangle illustrates the relationship between the three dimensions. **Content** is always influenced by the nature of the mental engagement arising from the incentive whether through necessity, intrigue or pleasure. **Incentive** is also influenced by the content with which the learning is concerned. **Interaction** influences sociality. Sociality is also influenced by the concerns and the content mobilised by those concerns because it develops via the acquistion process. Illeris asserts that only when all three dimensions are considered can a satisfactory quality of learning take place. Here the triangle is adapted to demonstrate the specific content, incentive and environment which are necessary for optimum reflection. The learner must understand and intuitively discern meaning in experience associating this with and accommodating it within what he already knows. This is the **content**. He must be willing to commit and engage honestly and openly with his environment aware of the part he plays in this. This is the **incentive**. In turn the environment must be conducive to peaceful contemplation within a generous time frame. In addition the environment should be populated with trusted others who participate in collaborative enquiry. This is **the environment**.

Figure 2.3   Illeris' tension triangle of learning

the tasks of living and working can become the reasons for working and living and reflection can be easily omitted from personal timetables by default. In a study of nursing work in an intensive care unit Stayt (2008) found that stored up emotion that was unacknowledged and unaddressed was detrimental to wellbeing. The significance of death and the way in which sharing the experience of loss with families intensified the nurse–patient relationship often resulted in cumulative grief. This outcome arose from the lack of time and opportunity to yield reflective space to loss leading to doubts about competency, loss of identity and low self-esteem. It is necessary then to purposefully schedule generous time out when planning to reflect (Welland and Bethune, 1996). In practice placement learners should negotiate time to reflect with practice teachers and practice teachers should be sympathetic to this (Billett, Smith and Barker, 2005). On campus this need is also rec- ognised. Reflections will also be richer and more productive when carried out in the company of others, but care should be taken that confidentiality and trust are established ground rules (Riley- Doucet and Wilson, 1997).

Encouraging individuality: avoiding prescribed narrative

Learners who produce reflective narratives which are judged as warranting improvement should *not* be asked to reproduce a second more detailed version. Guidance for improvement should be given with future narratives in mind. Requesting further editions of reflection on the same experience are an open invitation to the student to comply with pedagogy rather than behave as an independ- ent adult learner. Reflection should be spontaneous and shadow opportunistic discursive learning. Reflective narratives should not be 'made to order' or 'prescribed' to fit or prove competence in a certain domain of practice learning. Narratives whether written or as part of group discussion should follow student interest and purpose *and then* be used as additional evidence for the competencies or proficiencies to which they pertain. Prescribed reflection in practice risks forcing what should be spontaneous student centred behaviour and may produce a laboured disingenuous piece of work (Paterson, 1995; Richardson and Maltby, 1995).

Addressing the power relationship

Any teacher who employs reflection as a learning tool must also realise the *power relationship* that exists between the students and themselves. Students who are asked to declare their emotions and innermost thoughts may feel embarrassed and exposed. This 'power playing field' can be levelled by practice teachers who share their own reflective logs with their students openly admitting their own shortcomings and errors in the past and the present. This has been identified as one of the hall- marks of a good teacher (Greer, Pokorny, Clay, Brown and Steele, 2010).

Prescribed reflection in practice fails to take account of the additional mental and emotional workload it constitutes for a student already exhausted by the physical mental and emotional demands of long hours in a clinical setting (Welland and Bethune, 1996). Even in academia, assign- ments requiring reflection should supply clear guidelines linked to learning outcomes. The word limit margin should be wider and the submission deadline more flexible than in an essay to allow for individuality and diversity in expression and writing style.

Ethical considerations

Hargreaves (1997) has stressed the importance of ethical awareness in reflection. When we tell a story we have an ethical responsibility to represent the account as accurately and as fairly as we can. But this is just the beginning of ethical reflection. There is some overlap here with honesty in reflection in that we do not misrepresent others. Other people in the story are not aware that the story has been shared nor have they given their consent for us to publicise their involvement. The story is as we have perceived events to have taken place. It is our *claim* to the truth rather than the *absolute* truth. Others who populate our story have no opportunity to give their perspective. This obliges us to preserve the anonymity of those others but substituting a pseudonym for their real names and withholding other personal details that are irrelevant to the story. Note that in Table 2.1 Tony's address and the specifics of his clinical setting are not revealed.

Furthermore, we are able to tell our story because we are part of that story. We are not a passive observer in the way that someone would be if they were watching the account on film. We are active constituents of the story. Even if our role in the account involved doing nothing we were present in the situation. Therefore, we share an ethical responsibility to act, to address any morally questionable events within our account, raising them with the appropriate authority as soon as possible afterwards, especially if patients are involved (Rich and Parker, 1995).

The value of stories

Bruner (1999) has argued that stories have a special place in learning. Stories are knowledge and principles in the context of human existence. The knowledge stories contain is readily understood by us because it is embedded in the medium with which we best identify: life. We listen to a story for longer than we may study instructions in a manual or listen to a lecture in which we are 'talked at'. A story is a learning package which suspends our prejudices and holds our values up to questioning before we realise it while we absorb the point of view of the storyteller. Historically stories have been the means by which knowledge, values, beliefs, ethics and more have been inherited from and bequethed to successive generations. The teachings of the prophet Mohammed, the parables of Jesus Christ, the plays of William Shakespeare and writings of Charles Dickens are all examples of this. Narratives share a characteristic in that they usually involve a problem, disruptive element or central subject which requires addressing. Trouble can in this way be said to be 'the engine of narrative' or the font of ideas. Real life accounts should not be undervalued. As we shall see in the next chapter personal accounts enable history to be constructed, sociology to be argued and the future to be envisaged. Through the evidence they present real life accounts put theory to the test in practice; preserving or challenging existing values. Personal discourses also inform on the storytellers and are tools for understanding others. We may never truly understand the pain of bone metastases or appreciate the impact on mood until we hear the story of a sufferer.

Supplying external evidence

Knowing in the living, in the doing and from the doing is personally owned knowledge. It is part of a situation or series of situations we have experienced. It is *internal evidence. External evidence* is academically credible material on the subject matter central to your experience which serves to further inform on, support or challenge your own findings and conclusions. There is a wide range of evidence which can be used here. Avoid public information websites which will not supply you with the depth of knowledge you require. The best start is made by using an academic database search machine available online in any institute of higher education. Use three to six key words associated with the subject of your reflection and you will be provided with a plethora of peer reviewed papers which increase your understanding of research and theory pertaining to your experience. Expert guidance from charity websites and policy documents from government departments may also prove helpful. Textbooks and literature reviews are also very useful sources but the learner should take care to select the most recent material from this category. Professional codes of ethics from bodies such as the American Nurses Association or the Nursing and Midwifery Council of the United Kingdom can be used to support decisions.

A range of referenced academic sources within a reflective piece can look impressive but a word of caution is warranted. Many learners have been known to search academic databases until they find a paper which supports their own point of view arising from an experience. This is confirmation bias and should be avoided because it serves to narrow our field of knowledge rather than widen it. A piece of research selected purely because it tells us what we want to hear defeats the purpose of our reflection which is to broaden our understanding of an experience by exposing misconceptions, prejudices and assumptions and revealing our 'blind spots'.

Pursuing success in reflective practice

There are some key points to remember when striving to become reflective practitioner (Table 2.3). Formal learners in undergraduate or postgraduate study should make an early start in practising

Table 2.3 Tips for success

- Make an early start.
- Enjoy the informal dimension.
- Write things down – tidy up later.
- Remember your own ethical responsibilities.
- Carve out time in practice.
- Make use of 'passive time'.
- Share with academic tutor and practice teacher.
- The private and the public journals.
- Make study buddies.
- Share and swap evidence.

Table 2.4 The value of reflection to nursing practice

- Self-regulation.
- Prevention of complacency, ritual and habitualisation.
- Increases empathic ability.
- Increases self-awareness.
- Supplies freedom, growth and intuition in practice.

their reflective skills before other academic pressures crowd out time that might otherwise have been reserved for reflection. Despite the hectic pace of nursing life windows of passive time spent driving or on public transport still exist as part of a working day. These passive moments present solid opportunities for reflection which are less likely to be interrupted. There is a unique informal dimension to reflection which is there to be enjoyed. In the storytelling section of narrative, informal language can be used that would not be acceptable in an essay.

Expressions such as 'I could have punched the air when the patient thanked me and said that I had a very gentle touch' and 'I wanted to weep when I heard that my patient had attempted suicide again' are entirely appropriate because they capture the personal and individual experience of learning.

All nurses struggle with punishing schedules so whether reflection takes the form of journaling or reflecting in discussion brief contemporaneous notes should be taken to prevent ideas being lost. These can then be written up later if so desired. If journaling is the chosen method of reflection or a piece of reflective work as an assignment is being submitted it may be wise to keep a private journal from which text to be seen by others can be extracted. A support group of 'study buddies' reduces study time and aids sound reflection through the provision of a number of points of view. Within such a group evidence can also be swapped or shared.

The value to professional practice

When used properly and responsibly reflection is a valuable force for good in nursing practice. Reflection can help self-regulation by making us accountable to ourselves and presenting evidence of our continuing education to others. It is a tool with which to challenge any inconsistencies between what we practice and the value and belief systems we claim to espouse. Much of nursing practice can easily be viewed as a series of simple repetitive tasks and the inherent nursing skills at work can be invisible to patients and uninformed observers including nurses with a task orientated mentality. This can result in habitualisation: a state of complacency in which expert skills of experienced practice are minimised with the implication that they are common to everyone. The scrutiny which reflection requires works to prevent this. Reflection deconstructs and dissects the dynamics of an experience that may have appeared mundane while contemporaneous, but with evaluative hindsight may take on much deeper meaning. Repeated questioning of practice discourages nursing work from becoming a mere series of rituals which gives much more comfort to the practitioner than the patient and is divorced from any evidence base. The reflective practitioner is always trying to examine events through the eyes of others and is therefore well placed to develop the advanced empathic skills essential to quality patient-centred care and advocacy. As reflection also involves self-examination, it also has potential for greater self-awareness. This type of learning is needs led because it seeks to answer questions arising in practice as it happens. As such reflection supplies a knowledge and understanding of practice that helps develop expertise.

Conclusion

Reflection is way of thinking on our interpretation of experience to give it meaning; drawing on internal and external sources of knowledge. Reflection turns experience into learning. It can empower nurses to demonstrate accountability and self-regulation. Self-awareness, mindfulness, emotional intelligence, reflexivity, openness, honesty, creativity are all prerequisites for the individual. Peace and quiet, adequate ring fenced time and the company of trusted encouraging others are prerequisites of the environment. Teachers in practice and on campus need to give attention to the impact of power relationships and prescribed narrative on the genuineness of student learning. The absence of any one or more of these prerequisites will disable what is a fragile and personal process.

In this chapter we have introduced reflection as a basic concept and we have learned how to *demonstrate, describe and discuss* the learning that results from experience. Later in this book we will learn how to use *events* as tools for reflective learning. We will also begin to move beyond demonstration and description of learning toward *analysis.*

However, in the next chapter we pause to consider the place of reflection in professional life and judgement.

3 Why we need reflection

Box 3.1 Main points: Chapter 3

- The social world in which practitioners work is more complex and unpredictable than the natural world governed by laws of mathematics physics and chemistry which possess high levels of certitude.
- Interpretation and reflection are essential to move effectively in the social world.
- Reflection is not simply one source of knowing among many but a means of accessing all forms of knowledge.
- As a form of personal knowledge reflection as a human ability has a number of deficits but it is not fundamentally flawed.
- Artificial intelligence cannot comprehend the anomalies of the social world. It only works effectively in company with reflection and professional judgement.
- There are many forms of personal knowledge which prove reliable sources of evidence.

Introduction

We find that a lot of our senior house officers who come to the neonatal unit never having done neonatal before, after two months of having their feet under the table they think they know it all. Well actually, you know, they can learn from us and we do know what we are talking about. We can't always articulate it but then not all things can always be articulated. It is that instinctive, intuitive, it comes from experience. I can remember when I first started on neonatal 20 years ago; nurses would say that there is something wrong with a particular baby I would think 'well how do they know?'. I remember thinking: 'I wish I could be like that'. As experience comes you do learn to pick up what these feelings are. I think it is the same with any, whatever field of nursing you work in, I have got friends who work in adult intensive care and they can tell you the same kind of thing, that gut reaction, that gut feeling that you know something isn't quite right, even though you probably can't put your finger on it exactly.

(A charge nurse in neonatal intensive care)

Before we continue to develop our understanding of reflection and reflective practice we will pause briefly in this chapter to consider the place of reflection in human judgement. In a critique of Standing's Revised Continuum of Clinical Judgement and Decision Making in Nursing we will appraise the relationship between reflective practice and other forms of knowledge. A mental health nursing narrative will be used to illustrate a lived experience devoid of competent reflection. The value of propositional knowledge in the past and present will be critically compared with contemporary questions about the worth of reflection in professional life.

Life without reflection

Imagine if we could only experience a situation once and never grasp or benefit from its meaning. Imagine not being able to learn from experience; failing to capitalise on our successes or learn from our mistakes. Imagine having to use a guide book for everything including everyday tasks like brushing and flossing your teeth or cooking lunch. Picture a world where nobody was ever allowed to use their imagination, intuition or initiative. Imagine trying to solve a problem before first understanding what that problem was and not being able to relate one situation or one body of knowledge to another. Such an inability to seize and retain for ourselves personal ownership of knowledge of our world would be socially as well as intellectually disabling. We could not assess different forms of evidence and come to a reasoned decision. We could never examine the gaps in conversation and other unexplained silences, the facial expressions, body language and vocal tone, the sound and smells, the tastes and tactile messages that deliver information about an experience absent in the spoken word. Deprived of any chance to acquire acumen and develop life wisdom, our daily existence would be characterised by anxiety and bereft of any self-confidence. Working with others would be fraught with distrust if it were possible at all.

Paul Linsley's narrative (Box 3.2) about a young man with Schizophrenia provides us with a glimpse of what life would be like if we could not accurately reflect on our lives as we experience them. People such as 'Michael' who suffer from Schizophrenia cannot distinguish between their own thoughts and those of others. As such they can have no insight into their own state of being nor can they empathise with others. Fractured cognitive ability means that the vernacular and the pragmatic use of speech in the shape of methaphors, hints, humour, sarcasm and irony is unchartered territory for them. Hence they cannot discern the subtle indirect messages in language and this can be dispiriting if not frightening for them. Powers of perception used to comprehend events, judge propriety, sense danger, identify common ground with others and form bonds of trust and attachment are derailed. Furthermore people suffering from psychosis have no sense of agency or need to take personal responsibility in their lives. So when opportunities to learn or act on learning arise, they lack the motivation and initiative to benefit themselves from that learning. Furthermore, they cannot comprehend and theorise from any events they witness because they cannot construct a reliable cohesive narrative (Chan and Mak, 2012). In considering the disposition of 'Michael' and others like him we are exposed to the depersonalised and impoverished life experience that would be ours if not for our ability to reflect on our experience; sifting through the emotions, actions and decisions that issue from that experience; being 'present' in the moment and making extemporaneous judgements in the face of unanticipated events as they have meaning for the self and others.

Box 3.2   'Michael'

By Paul Linsley, RMHN

I'm glad Michael's parents were here to meet me. I don't think Michael would have let me into the house otherwise. Despite his illness, Michael trusts his parents. It is clear that he's unwell, he looks unkempt and has difficulty concentrating on what I'm asking him? He seems suspicious of me and repeatedly asks what I am doing here.

Michael has had a history of continuous schizophrenia for 4 years. He is preoccupied with delusions and suffers frequent auditory hallucinations. Despite this he lives independently with the support of his family and attends the local day centre; however, his attendance at the centre has been erratic of late, and he has not been for the last week.

Although he is seated he seems to be on edge. His eyes are darting around the room and he is clearly suspicious of my being here. His parents believe that he's not been taking his medication, although they have no evidence to support this. I feel sorry for them, they clearly love their son and are distressed to see him unwell. There is no history of mental illness in the family and this is something that they've had to learn to cope with.

Michael says that he's not slept 'for a number of nights'. He says that he's afraid to sleep because he's frightened that someone might break into his house and set him alight. His speech is becoming more pressured as he tries to get his words out and I have trouble keeping up with what he has to say. I ask him why someone would want to do him harm? He becomes quite agitated at this. Stuttering, Michael explains that he smells. Can't I smell him? He says that he smells of rotting fish and cabbages. The fumes from him stink. They are so pungent 'that if someone lit a match then he could blow up a house'.

Without warning he leaps out of his chair making me and his parents jump. Talking about his thoughts seems to have distressed him as he looks close to tears. He looks at me as if trying to weigh me up and then bursts into a fit of giggles.

'Smelly pants, smelly pants, arse on fire. Even the Queen farts. Put a cork up my arse that'll stop the smell escaping. Nobody light a match!' he screams.

His speech is becoming more rapid and disinhibited. His mum has started to cry, Michael's dad seeks to comfort her. I try to focus and respond to Michael's mood as his speech is now so disorganised that I can no longer hold a conversation with him. I try to act in a calm manner and encourage Michael to sit and collect himself. Instead he takes himself off to a corner of the room where he stands in silence pressing his bottom against the wall apparently in an effort to stop himself from breaking wind.

It is clear that the assessment is going to take some time.

These faculties are so embedded in the fabric of everyday life that we are seldom conscious of them unless we are engaged in higher learning or are harnessing reflection for some deliberate discursive praxis. Nevertheless this everyday social competence is essential for negotiating the complex world in which we live and work.

The nature of the social world

The social world is the world inhabited by sentient human beings as they interpret and construct it. In this world nothing has meaning until meaning is attributed to it by a conscious being. Material bodies may exist but this is not the same as being interpreted as having meaning. Objects are what distinguish dreams and fabrications from real life interpretations. This contrasts with the natural world which is governed by scientific laws and where events can be predicted through mathematical calculation and observation of the laws of physics and chemistry. Certitude in the natural world is not ubiquitous but it is much more common than in the social world. In the social world certitude proves elusive because of the different possibilities arising from diversity in human interpretation and behaviour (Crotty, 1998). The range of interpretation is dependent upon a person's experience and expertise, ignorance and prejudice, values and culture. The environment in which people move and exist also provides a diverse vault of variables which impact on events and behaviour. Consequently, at any time and place the number of anomalies, contingencies, exit and entrance points in any stream of events is infinite. Experience and the object of experience are inseparable, as are the interpretation from the experience and the object from the conscious interpretation. From this perspective objectivism and subjectivism are polarised oversimplifications of reality (Lincoln and Guba, 2000). The reality of knowledge and discovery is more precisely reflected in the interaction of object and conscious interpreter (Lotman, 1990). This interaction is called situated cognition. Situated cognition is the point from which judgement takes place (Stake, 2000).

Judgement and decision making for the social world

The complexity of the social world requires that professional judgement is a multifaceted exercise. This is implied by Standing (2008: 125) who defines judgment as 'the assessment of alternatives regarding possible causes of action and decision making; the management of uncertainty about problems encountered, alternative solutions available and a persons ability to cope'.

Standing's continuum of judgement and decision making (Figure 3.1) illustrates the range of forms of knowledge which is resourced in nursing judgement and decision making. On the right the continuum ranges from randomised controlled trials with a high level of demonstrable rigor through quantative and qualitative research to action research and audit. On the far left of the continuum are forms of personal or propositional knowledge so called because they are subject to bias and are more open to question than knowledge confirmed by structured scientific methods. Cognitive modes on the left hand side of the table form a picture of the autonomous practitioner who draws on the knowledge of experience to respond to clinical need for which they stand accountable. Propositional knowledge includes intuition; 'the ability to perceive or know things without conscious reasoning' (Lawrence, 2012: 5). Intuitive knowledge enables pattern recognition and relating wholes to the parts of experience and vice versa (Benner and Tanner, 1987; Benner, Tanner and Chesla, 1996). Intuition also involves embodied knowledge through the knowing in the doing discussed in Chapter 2. Reflection also sits in this category because it is knowledge induced from the interpretation of experience and therefore personally owned. Peer aided judgement or collaborative enquiry is also a form of propositional knowledge because it arises from peer exploration discussion and debate of a subject.

Standing's continuum while helpful in the demarcation of judgement modes confines mixed methods of thinking to quasi-rationality (pictured in the middle of the chart). In this it does not do justice to the flexibility and complexity of the human brain. Talk of 'tasks requiring different modes of thinking' (Standing, 2008: 127) means that no account is taken of the 'hybrid' styles of thinking *across* the continuum and this is misleading. Klein (2001) casts doubt over the reality of any barrier between 'hard' and 'soft' science by declaring that intuitive thinking is behind many of the decisions taken in rigorously controlled laboratory trials. Furthermore, the scientist in the laboratory must interpret and reflect on the implications of his findings. In fact, many of the great fathers of science such as Thomas Edison followed 'hunches' (Carlson and Kaiser, 1999). Moreover, practitioners frequently reflect on their practice with the application of both quantitative and qualitative research findings in mind (Almond, 2001; Wilson and Crowe, 2008).

Interpretation and reflection have a part to play in any form of knowledge judgement and decision making. It seems that the reflective practitoner is able to simultaneously use a combination of formal knowledge (research findings, evidence based guidance, professional ethics and values) and informal knowledge (intuitive recognition of patterns and relationships along with common sense understanding borne from experience) to navigate their way with effect in practice (Benner, 1987; Benner, Tanner and Chesla, 1996; Almond, 2001; Wilson and Crowe, 2008). Schon (1987) asserted that professional assessment and diagnosis are two separate phases of practice arguing that problems do not present themselves in an organised way but are often hidden in a 'mess' of different forms of information. Diagnosis is the framing or defining of the object of practitioner attention; the end result of assessment which is the structuring and prioritising of events, problems and other characteristics of the practice scene. This uniquely human and extremely flexible approach to the social world means that practitioners are able to act with contingency; 'thinking on their feet' in the face of the irregular and unexpected in the practice landscape. They are able to mentally 'revisit' a prior practice scene to explore decision making and make recommendations for future best practice. This explains the central place of reflection in nursing practice: the need to make sense of the ambigious mess that is the social world in which we live and work (Schon, 1987; Hannigan, 2001). However, this position is not without its deficits and its critics.

Boud (2010) points out the extent to which reflection and journals of reflection have been misused in education within rigid and suppressive rules and guidelines which fail to acknowledge the highly fragile and individual shape of the process. This includes the denial of students the time space and solitude to adequately reflect on experience (Welland and Bethune, 1996) and overlooking ethical concerns about intrusion on privacy and the consequences of 'emotional fallout' (Rich and Parker, 1995). Attention has also been drawn to problems with the cognitive process at the heart of reflection. For example memory plays a crucial role despite evidence raising questions about its reliability. The tendency among human beings to simplify and reduce information to make it more manageable would appear to be partly responsible for this (Talbot, 2012). Much reflective practice contains the implication that all the constituents of an experience are predictable and that the 'lessons' of such 'failure' to anticipate events can be transferred to other similar situations. Such 'hindsight bias' is misleading as practice and social life are heavily influenced by time and circumstance which defy prediction and anticipation (Jones, 1995: 783). Self-justification and the perceived need to address cognitive dissonance have been shown to take priority over the search for meaning in experience. This partners confirmation bias in which

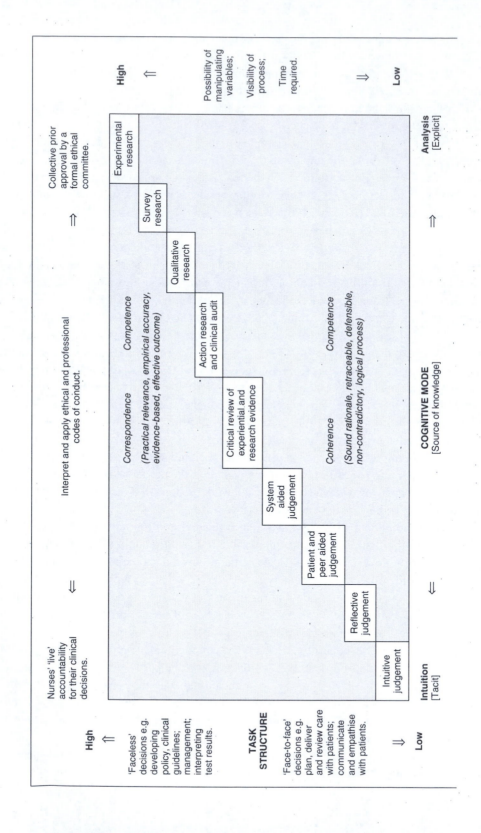

Standing's cognitive continuum (Standing, 2008) illustrates the range of modes involved in clinical judgement. The horizontal axis illustrates the different ways of sourcing knowledge. The vertical axis illustrates the level of reliability set against the context of the task at hand and the time required to use the mode. The left hand side of the table houses forms of thinking used 'in the moment' which operate without conscious access to formal scientific knowledge. These judgement modes are associated with human ability to adapt and survive through social learning in changing situations. This is personally owned or propositional knowledge. The right hand side of the table leans toward knowledge built on logic, mathematics and the application of computer technology to factor in predictability within judgement. In experimental research involving randomised controlled trials the impact of an intervention (usually a treatment) on one group is examined in comparison with an identical group that does not receive the intervention. The results are seen as possessing a high level of reliability and validity because the risk of human bias is minimised. However, while the method is suitable for clinical trials involving medication or some psychiatric interventions, it does not discern the lived experience of the participant; only an observed result. Furthermore the use of a control group has limited value in social research because of the unpredictable influence of human motives and values. Quantitative research systematically tests and describes relationships to explore cause and effect through the use of statistics. The strength of quantitative research is describing what is happening but not why it is happening. For example a quantitative study may tell us that less people in a particular country are smoking now than 10 years ago in line with a national ban on advertising and smoking in public places. However, the precise reasons as to why there are more ex-smokers themselves have not been asked. Quantative methods used in a survey may obtain some of the answers but because the questions are fixed the participants have no opportunity to declare or discuss what is important to them. On the other hand qualitative research enquires into the meaning of life experiences through the provision of structured description and analysis of declarative knowledge. The method seeks to lend rigor and reliability to the collection of personally owned information but while its findings may have implications for other settings they can not be generalised in the same way as the impact of a drug in a clinical trial. They are context specific. Action research and clinical audit, while still on the right of the continuum sit closer to the middle because they seek to test applied evidence base criteria in a fixed social setting (Grove, Burns and Gray, 2013). Overall the larger an active part is played by human beings and the social world the less reliable and rigorous the decision making mode is deemed to be. Intuition and reflection sit on the far left of the table because they describe knowledge owned by the individual. Intuition is knowledge recalled from memory as a result of a perceived sense of salience in response to stimuli from the special sense centres. Intuitive knowledge enables pattern recognition and relating the whole to the parts of an experience and vice versa (Benner and Tanner, 1987; Benner, Tanner and Chesla, 1996). It is 'the ability to perceive or know things without conscious reasoning' (Lawrence, 2012: 5). Reflection and intuition are closely related. When an experience is 'revisited' mental landmarks are pitched which link neural matrices with all five special senses (Benner and Tanner 1987, Schon 1987). When, in the course of future practice, these landmarks are alerted by the occurrence of similar episodes, they code for delivery of pre-packaged information which allow the nurse to grasp the situation directly without time-costly prior consideration (Benner and Tanner, 1987; Appleton and King, 1997). Furthermore reflection on the basis for intuitive knowing aids articulation of how we know. In these ways intuitive practice is greatly enhanced by reflection and reflection helps develop expertise. Peer aided judgement sits further toward the right on the table because the number of participants reduces the chance of error and increases validatory power. System aided judgement such as that arising from the use of a clinical pathway of care or from a systematic review of literature is closer toward the right because it involves clinical research findings but remains on the left side of the table because it is knowledge which is being personally applied in practice life. The intuitive end of the continuum is characterised by frequent but relatively small errors. The analytical end is characterised by infrequent but sizeable errors such as false positives and false negatives in screening programmes such as those offering cervical smears or mammography.

Figure 3.1   Standing's revised continuum of clinical judgement and decision making in nursing: nine modes of practice

the student will search only for evidence which supports their existing views or performs a complaint academic study task which tells their lecturer or practice teacher what they believe they want to hear (Talbot, 2012). Introspection bias in which the learner has an exaggerated view of their own objectivity in relation to that of others, also threatens the validity of reflection (Pronin and Kugler, 2006). However, despite this, human reflection still compares well with artificial intelligence in a variety of forms.

The limits of artificial intelligence

No human intellectual activity is perfect but neither is it usually incompetent (Polanyi, 1998). Personal knowledge such as records of lived experience, intuitive judgement and reflection while not infallible have some advantages over artificial intelligence units such as pathways and protocols based on disembodied scientific evidence. Structured systematic analysis is time consuming. Reflection and intuition are swift and frequently accurate within safe boundaries (Standing, 2008). Artificial intelligence units seek to impose disembodied research evidence on an environment they assume is identical to the one in which the research was conducted. This is a significant weakness. On the other hand, human beings are not passive recipients of information who respond to stimuli in predictable ways. They are not mere carriers or managers and manipulators of information in the way that an electronic system might be defined. Humans are interpretors and creators, equipped to respond flexibly and imaginatively to the challenges of practice. Artificial intelligence units are pre-programmed to react and address certain fixed templates. Beyond this context there is no meaning for such units. The symbols which trigger a response from a computer system have no unified meaning for the computer. Computated actions always follow programming. Robotic pathways carry no evaluative component and have no way of discerning a language system rendered inadequate by a changing environment. Neither can such units discern the different meanings and senses supplied to the same word by context. On the contrary they continue to perform as programmed (Bredo, 1999). Artificial intelligence units (AIU) have no 'common sense understanding' with which to embrace the wholeness of a matter with all its anomalies. They cannot pause to reconsider or reflect in the face of new information or unforeseen circumstances which may serve to mitigate or alter action as required. AIU cannot have empathy or discern changes in human behaviour. This is the frequent source of frustration for nurses who must work with systems which do not possess human insight.

We are often given the impression that artificial intelligence or imposed guidance and directives give us our understanding of our world addressing the deficits in human judgement. In fact the relationship between artificial intelligence and human judgement is much more of an equal partnership. Both have deficits. Attempts to apply rules originating in the more predictable natural world (logical positivism) to the social world rarely meet with any level of success (Bredo, 1999) as shown in the narrative of a nurse in charge of a substance misuse clinic (Box 3.3). Artificial intelligence, imposed guidance and directives are impotent without the human judgement they are designed to assist. In nursing life this is evident in the use of clinical pathways and other evidence based guidance. For example Appleton and Cowley (2004) found that the use of evidence based guidance for the identification of vulnerable families produced many false positives when health visitors' contextual knowledge of their communities was brought to bear on assessment. Alternatively local contextual knowledge meant that community practitioners were often concerned about families who did not register with official vulnerability criteria. Research has also shown that the Liverpool Care Pathway cannot ensure the optimum end of life care it was designed to promote without effective team communication (Messam and Pettifer, 2009), judicious professional monitoring of its application (Preston, 2007) or the provision of emotional intelligence and compassionate care (Murphy, 2011).

Box 3.3   The trouble with standards and targets

You know sometimes I wish some people would come and live in the real world – they come in here, they observe practice, they ask questions and yes, they listen to the answers. But they don't always seem to get the 'human element' in our work. Our unit is always busy but it is not just about how many nurses are caring for how many patients and for how long. If that were all there was to it the job would be much simpler. No one can guarantee what comes through our door whether the appointment is scheduled or unscheduled. But you *can* guarantee what we expect or what we have been told in advance isn't going to match what we get. There are *always* complications: from infected injection sites to patients going off; from social problems which present out of the blue to relatives and carers who need help themselves. And so there are implications for nursing practice there. Unexpected complications require unexpected and previously unplanned care and referral . . . and it all takes time and expert effort. We can't just say 'Hey . . . I'm so sorry but I have other people I need to see!'. People can tell when you don't want to listen or when you're not interested. We have known some of these patients and their families for years and you can never tell when you might see some of the new ones again. Working on the back of these relationships is what moves care, recovery and rehabilitation forward. And if we neglect time needed to listen and be there for these people we may well succeed in meeting one set of standards but we would certainly be failing to meet another.

So yes . . . 'on paper' if you reduced the length of time for each patient slot in each area then we would be able to see more patients in less time and theoretically people would be seen quicker. But in the real world these rigid ideas go 'out of the window' before you can even think about applying them. And you are faced with more chaos and more stress for everyone when you try.

We all like to do a good job around here. We care about the people we look after and we think it shows. So by all means let's have standards and let's set ourselves targets but for heavens sake let's make them realistic and reachable. And if we don't always meet them let's understand why.

(A nurse in charge of a combined addiction and substance misuse clinic)

Humans exist in a world of situated cognition where 'a situation in which an expression is used helps disambiguate a situation' (Bredo, 1999: 36). Humans possess common sense understandings which balance prescribed guideline pathways, protocol directives and recommendations for categorised situations against the unique variations of those situations. They are able to supply context to the interaction between evidence based guidance and the additional information emerging from contextualised behaviour and the contingent responses they require.

Through their interaction with their world their thoughts, actions and very being are refined by the world and by their own entrances. Speakers reflect on their speech and amend it (Standish, Smeyers and Smith, 2006), artists are continually refining their art in progress (Laurence, 2012) and writers are moulded by their reflections on their written work (Bredo, 1999). How many times have we changed what we have written in an email before we finish writing it? This situation of perpetual exchange explains why a persons beliefs and values are not always consistent with their actions.

The power of personal knowledge

Personal or propositional knowledge as evidence takes many forms (Box 3.4). Personal knowledge can be tainted by bias and prejudice but it may also be corrected by ethical awareness and caring. Its imperfections have never prevented the police and the courts using it in large measure to help convict, dismiss or acquit individuals suspected or accused of crime. Many eye witnesses have remained robust in court in the face of scrupulous cross examination by barristers using methods fuelled by the very evidence utilised by critics of reflection. When expert witnesses are called to court they are required to demonstrate that their interpretation and application of scientific evidence is valid. However, often the scientific evidence they use is also questioned as to its reliability and fitness for application. On the other side of the judicial process, Pennington and Hastie (1986; 1988) have shown how jurors sift information of different types and quality; forming theory like the assembling of a jigsaw to create a cohesive probable narrative. At each juncture the ubiquitous role of interpretation and reflection in accessing evidence is recognised.

Box 3.4   Examples of propositional knowledge as evidence

- Eye witness accounts and testimonies.
- Expert opinion.
- Autobiographies.
- Letters.
- Diaries.
- Reflective journals.
- Minutes of meetings.

The subjective nature of letters diaries and minutes from the past has not prevented them being hailed as historical artefacts and used by historians to construct history (Bruner, 1999). Propositional knowledge in the form of eye witness testimony for all its acknowledged flaws has also proved reliable when standing in opposition to scientific judgement. For many years, survivors of the Titanic sinking insisted that the ship broke in half as it sunk. Structural marine engineers claimed this was impossible in a ship of the Titanic's size. Yet when the wreck was eventually found eye witness testimony was validated.

So rather than be concerned about the feasibility of reflection as a tool for learning we need to be concerned about the ground rules and principles such as honesty, creativity, time, space and collaborative enquiry negotiated with students in advance of its use. Students need to understand the importance of reflexivity which cannot truly be falsified, at least not with any benefit to the falsifier. We also need to be concerned with the acceptance within assessment of the expressed informal personal and individual dimensions which would not be acceptable in other more traditional academic work. The imperfection of human judgement needs to be acknowledged but so do its strengths and unparalleled flexibility. The usefulness of scientific knowledge and evidence based tools to nursing practice cannot be underestimated but the role of professional judgement and reflection in accessing and deploying all forms of knowledge must also be respected.

Conclusion

Reflection and interpretation are central to human learning, judgement and decision making in the social world in which nurses practice. Contemporary personal knowledge in nursing can no more be devalued than the many forms it takes in the hands of eye witnesses, lawyers, jurors, judges and historians.

However, as reflection takes place within each person's own frame of reference, memory and culture which introduce bias how can these be minimised? This question will be addressed in Chapters 5 and 6. In the next chapter, however, we will examine the potential for learning in singular events.

4 Critical incidents

> ## Box 4.1   Main points: Chapter 4
>
> - Critical incidents are significant events that help us re-evaluate some aspects of life.
> - They can be positive or negative.
> - They are sometimes called 'lightbulb moments' because of the way we come to a certain new point of learning suddenly.
> - They harness the way our brain manages information in an 'associative' way.
> - They help us realise that the routine parts of life are unusual.
> - They are valuable sources of innovation and should be shared with others.

This chapter will define and explore critical incidents and their value to practice. The terms 'critical incident' and 'significant event' will be used interchangeably. We will draw on educational psychology and neural theories of learning to explain the nature and function of critical incidents as distinct from other forms of reflective activity. Narratives relating to significant turning points in individual learning will also be resourced and discussed. A guide to analysing a critical incident is provided.

Definition and history

A critical incident (sometimes called a significant event) is a happening which is deemed significant by the person who experiences it in that it opens a window of opportunity for critical evaluation of some aspect of life. It is set apart from the rest of reflective activity in that no search for meaning is required. The event is perceived as sufficiently inspirational so that meaning is apprehended swiftly, often instantaneously (Tripp, 1992). For this reason it is often referred to as a 'lightbulb moment' because of the accelerated way in which new knowledge is personally owned. However, the individual nature of the experience may mean that the meaning may be obvious only to the person who owns it.

Critical incidents were first coined and explored by Flanagan (1954) who identified turning points in military strategy through the eyes of war veterans. Strategists were able to identify key events which were by themselves influential on the flow and direction of other events and the actions of other individuals. These key events invariably revealed skills, knowledge, approaches, and attitudes that may not have been previously realised and therefore had not been shared. Flanagan's critical incident technique has been adopted across a range of professions seeking continuous improvement in their practice.

Flanagan (1954: 327) defined a critical incident as:

> any observable human activity that is sufficiently complete in itself to permit inferences and predictions to be made about the person performing the act. To be critical an incident must occur in a situation where the purpose or intent of the act seems fairly clear to the observer and where its consequences are sufficiently definite to leave little doubt concerning its effects.

In this context incidents are seen as critical not because they are necessarily negative but because of the pivotal role or 'tipping point' they have in learning. Critical incidents may present the essential challenge or critique to pre-existing patterns of thought and behaviour. On the other hand such an incident may well endorse current thinking and practice by providing fresh evidence of its worth or highlighting some aspect of good practice which has hitherto gone unacknowledged and can be shared with others. Significant events essentially help individuals to see a fresh aspect to something already well known to them.

For the learner in a nursing setting there are a range of reasons why it is important to think of critical incidents as positive experiences. Nursing has historically existed in a very self-critical even denigrating environment in which weaknesses are often highlighted over strengths. Crowe (2000) speaks of this environment as being built on traditional values which view caring as the natural activity of any 'good' woman. This value base fails to discern caring as having an independent epistemology which produces expertise in practice. A disproportionate preoccupation with modesty, subservience and altruism as womanly virtues and achievement and creativity as working in opposition to these virtues has served to stifle the celebration and advertising of success in caring arts and sciences. Professional jealousy and resistance to change also work a inhibitive influence on innovation and creativity suppressing and undermining ideas and practices which seek to forge better ways of working. Many information gathering systems aimed at measuring quality ignore records of excellence in practice designed as they are to monitor errors and omissions seen as central to risk management. It is important that practitioners do not allow such a restrictive professional culture to prevent them from focusing on and publishing their strengths as well as their deficits. While it is true that much learning arises from making mistakes, this type of experience can be a painful teacher. Used exclusively shared negative experiences can reap regret shame and embarrassment. They can be alarmist and produce decisions which are built on disproportionate fear and anxiety. This in turn can result in a workforce burdened down with warnings. A positive experience on the other hand can be joyful in that it provides the realisation of getting something right or doing something well. Sharing the principles arising from positive experiences also shares a feeling of joy and produces decisions which are built on confidence and optimism. This can produce a satisfied workforce that is inspired and imaginative. As adult participants in life long learning we each have a rich, diverse life database from which to act intuitively and creatively only realising so when alerted by some related event.

Critical incidents have certain characteristics:

1. They are mental cues.
2. They present a snapshot of practice life.
3. They reveal the fiction of the untoward.
4. They represent an irrational intuitive way of thinking.

We will examine each of these characteristics one at a time.

Mental cues: neural perspectives on critical incidents

The way our brains manage information; the neural kinetics and dynamics of memory and attention together with the role of emotion as a thought trigger lend support to the semantic nature of feeling, learning and knowing. We feel, learn and know as it has personal meaning for us. More specifically neural architecture explains the mechanism pertaining to critical incidents. Longterm memory does not exist as a distinct specialised centre but as an associative matrix: a multiple state entity networked across centres by which information is stored through relationship with personal meaning and context. So although our life roles may be well defined, our life experience as represented in our brains is seamless. Neural networks crosslink in terms of their hierarchical and comparative relationships. Networks also have an activational spread which is linked to the sensory mode(s) of the stimuli (visual (what we see), tactile (what we touch), auditory (what we hear), olfactory (what we smell) and gustatory (what we taste)) which trigger the retrieval of information (Cohen, 1993). Essentially, the ability of external cues to retreive information is dependent not on raw data but on perceived salience and personal meaning (Tulving and Schacter, 1990). The smell of a particular food may remind us of an enjoyable gathering with friends. The sound of certain music may instantly recall to our minds events and people we thought we had long forgotten. Perceived salience is also well illustrated in word association. For example the word 'blind' might be interpreted as the shade cover for a window rather than the description of one who has no sight. A sense of salience is also evident in a person's ability to recall their situation on 11 September 2001 but inability to recall their situation on the day prior to that date (unless something significant happened then too!). The semantic association in the 'stockhold' of memory moulds future attention and associated behaviours (Humphreys et al., 2003). Cohen (1993: 390) calls this the 'semantic relatedness effect'. This neural network in which memory and attention are interweaved explains the ability of a person to form a relationship between two situations which in any realm of attempted objectivity or third party attendance do not seem related at all. This is tangential thought; thinking which veers off at a tangent.

The catalyst for tangential reasoning is affect but an examination of the collage of evidence reveals this to be an oversimpified explanation. Polanyi (1998) has argued that passions, the fear and excitement of suspicion, the elation of discovery, cannot be separated from the thoughts they drive and the deeds and achievements they generate. Memories are 'tagged' with certain emotions so experiencing these emotions again stimulates the related memories. This is what makes critical incidents work for us. Tangential thought is possible because of the commonality of an emotion experienced across a range of experiences. This is called affective generic particularity. While the power of narrative exists to convey one human condition to another, before this happens a person is able to make a bridge between one experience and another because of the conscious emotions those experiences share. Knowledge is a feeling state because emotion acts as a 'rudder' for our perception and judgement. We feel before we think (Immordino and Damassio, 2007: 6). Strongly experienced but unexplored emotions deserve our interest and enquiry as they exist to stimulate our awareness of unacknowledged meaning. The value of emotions to reflection and judgement will be discussed in detail in Chapter 8.

We may think that we have never experienced a critical incident. But in view of these neural insights on memory, emotion and learning, we need to think again! It is likely that everyday all of us experience 'something that reminds us or makes us think differently about something else'. Epiphanies, a disagreement with someone, a dilemma or crisis, a defeat or a victory, a surprise or shock or any situation which results in us experiencing a strong emotion are all significant events. Stories, pictures, music and songs set or played out against a backdrop which is meaningful to us are also powerful catalysts for critical incidents. Indeed most episodes of learning have a critical point at which 'the penny drops' (Boud, Keogh and Walker, 1985).

Critical incidents as 'snapshots'

Critical incidents have been called 'snapshots' of life and practice (Clamp, 1979). However, the photography metaphor is potentially misleading and has more depth than may appear on initial consideration. It is not meant to imply a mere motionless and one dimensional reproduction of a moment in time. Such a reproduction might misrepresent more than it accurately conveys. A photograph carries more than visual knowledge to the viewer. A photograph will trigger a wide range of personal meanings of an emotive, social, psychological, cultural and cognitive nature. The context of a family photograph and the relationships therein portrayed or implied may deliver much more data than the visual image in isolation; the individuals, the expressed behaviours, the landscape, the style of dress together with the time period inferred (Box 4.2). All are separate interwoven strands of information which can initiate critical thinking and evaluation. In fact, the nature of such thinking means that it is impossible to isolate such visual information from the unique interpretation which the individual will place on it. It is in this latter sense that a critical incident is a 'snapshot'.

Box 4.2 A photograph as a critical incident

Today when I was in the attic I found a picture of myself with my son when he was 6 years old. We are pictured eating ice-cream on the beach. First I was taken by how much I had aged and how yesterday's fashions can sometimes look drab or even absurd and extreme today. But then I began to look more closely. I had forgotten what a handsome and carefree child James had been at that age.

Moreover, we look so happy. The thing I remember most about that holiday is not the places we visited, the things we did or the money we spent. It is our laughter. Everyday we seemed to have something to laugh about and the closeness of our relationship was visible for anyone to see. How different all this is from the way we are today. How can it be that we do not even speak to each other anymore? How did this happen? Where did it start?

A misguided sense of priorities caused me to stop listening to James when he reached adolescence and I would always overreact to his opinions when they differed from my own. When he started self-harming my attempts to help must have seemed to him more like interrogation than support. I talked too much, listened too little and gave up far too early. Love is often hardest to give to our children when they need it most. And then when we realise what we should have done it's often too late.

James is now a grown man. I am proud of the place he has made for himself in the world but he does not know this. What is more, I have never stopped to think about our relationship or my role in its deterioration until now. He means more to me than anything else in my life so why haven't I told him? It is as if I wrote him out of my world and can't find a way of writing him back in again. Can I really be such a fool to have valued my pride over a relationship with my son? I have said and done so many things that cannot be taken back or undone, but surely I can apologise or somehow work towards making amends.

It's strange what looking at an old photograph can do for you!

The fiction of the untoward

We tend to think of the untoward or unexpected as unusual and the routine as the norm. It would seem that the opposite is true. Benner (1984) argued that critical incidents expose the fiction of the untoward. The reality of professional life is revealed as an unfolding tapestry whose complex designs, visions and illustrations are challenging and fulfilling because of the unforseen nature of their shape and existence. Routine experiences can be described as such only with hindsight and even then only because they have been experienced as segments of meaning many times over. A 'routine' delivery by a midwife is one that is over. A 'routine' home visit by a community nurse is one that has passed. A 'routine' assessment is one that is complete. Cowley (1995) demonstrated this in the context of community nursing in a large qualitative study. Breadth and depth of expertise was shown to enable practitioners prepared for one particular scenario to shift the focus of practice away from predetermined objectives to address more pressing needs which had been hidden until the time of the episode of care. Cowley concluded that 'routine' was an inappropriate term which oversimplified the practice situation and devalued the skills necessary to operate effectively within it. Modern healthcare employs clinical pathways and protocols in an attempt to factor in predictability in practice, but such tools only function in partnership with clinical judgement to discern the measure of intervention, and when deviation from protocol is required (Peate, 2006). Management of the unpredictable requires humanity. It is this very feature of unpredictability in practice which makes it fertile ground for uncovering ingenuity and innovation arising from unforeseen occurrence.

The nature of critical incident: thinking and learning

The thinking which powers the exploitation of critical incidents is not rational. It is tangential and intuitive valuing situated cognition; a perspective couched in the values of 'Gestalt' (Figure 4.1); the world as an individual sees the world. The incident and the subject of reflection which issues forth from it share a concept valued by the individual. Through this 'concept translation', new knowledge is discovered. It is something we are helped to appraise via thinking about something else. Voluntary engagement by a practitioner in critical incident analysis therefore holds rich promise in terms of its potential for positive change not only in like situations but in other areas of practice which at first glance may seem to bear no relation to the event under consideration. However, a relationship *does* exist via the values or behaviour made transparent by some unexpected event (Cioffi, 1997). In education, teachers may attempt to plan or construct critical incidents. Through use of a range of techniques and in the shape of any number of surprises they may try to engineer tangential and transformative thought in their students. Audio and/or visual material can be used to 'jump start' a learner's thinking in a certain direction but this may not be to that learner's taste and the 'lesson' may backfire. Instead of finding the event significant for the right reason the student may find such an engineered event irritating, offensive, boring or inappropriately humorous. The existential nature of the phenomena means that outcomes cannot be predicted and such strategies carry varying degrees of risk. So there is need for caution. It is the student, not the teacher who must determine what is significant. Critical incidents begin with learner not the teacher.

Significant events stimulate us to move beyond our usual world. They disrupt our plans and assumptions. Narratives of life exist as consious theory in the mind long before they are written down (if in fact they ever are). They are the means by which we give structure to our goals and enshrine our achievements. Critical incidents are immediate prominences on the topical landscape of experience because they disrupt our plans and fragment our assumptions. Like all narratives for reflection critical incidents are examples of the 'trouble' which Jerome Bruner (1999: 99) calls the 'engine of narrative'. This engine is what drives us onwards but also upwards. Strategies for focusing on subsidiary awareness are important to hone our skills and optimise practice. Strategies for focusing on values underpinning our practices are important to promote justice as well as efficacy. The tangential pathway of thinking supplied by critical incidents is essential. Without it, the content of our secure contextualised world would never be disturbed. Critical incidents alert the mind to a

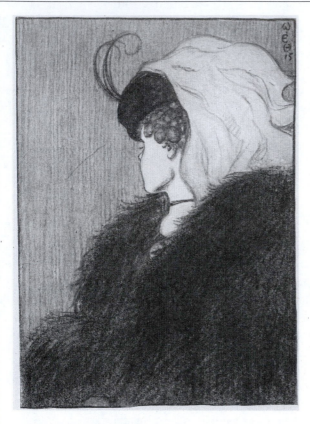

'Gestalt' is a psychological phenomenon which captures the notion of the uniqueness of each individual interpretation of the same object, group of objects or situation. Gestalt theory argues that we see our world, not as mere lines, shapes and shades of colour but in an organised state as it has meaning for us. Look at the picture on the left. It is a well known drawing called 'My wife and my mother in law'. The artist is said to have noticed his mother in law approaching while he was sketching a portrait of his young wife. But who did he draw in the end? Was it his wife looking over her right shoulder or his mother in law: a hideous 'witch like' hooded figure?

Images of both are contained within the portrait. Which do you find easier to see? Is it the young woman or her mother? Do you find it easier to see the young woman? The young woman's cheek and jaw line is also the old woman's large hooked nose and the young woman's ear is the old woman's left eye. The young woman's neckline is the old woman's chin.

Do you find it easier to see the old woman? The old woman is portrayed laterally facing to her right while the young woman is looking over her right shoulder. The old woman's thin lips are the young woman's choker necklace. The old woman's right eye is the young woman's eye lash and nose.

The portrait presents a puzzle for the mind, revealing how differently we may all interpret the same visual information because of the diversity in our vault of values and experience. Gestalt theory lends support to the value of critical incidents. A positive or negative event may highlight the importance of a particular feature of our lives which will be completely insignificant to someone else also exposed to the same event. We interpret situations and experiences as they have meaning for us.

Figure 4.1 Gestalt theory

higher plain of principles beyond the daily practice of life, helping us to revisit situations and practices in a more informed way.

Exploring and comparing critical incidents

Joanna Pilarska 's experience (Box 4.3) is a true 'light bulb moment'. It is worth noting that at least some of the theory she discusses in relation to Edna was already known to her. It took this event to 'bring the meaning home' making real to her words and concepts she thought she had already understood in lectures and background reading. As we read Pilarska's discourse we are made aware of the proclivity to make prior judgements in our daily lives and the need to suspend these in the course of practice.

Box 4.3   The lady in the green armchair

By Joanna Pilarska

Whilst on community placement I met a patient called Edna. Edna is an eighty-four-year-old lady who has been suffering from diabetes, heart disease, obesity and venous leg ulcerations for many years. My practice teacher and I visited Edna twice a week to change the dressings on both of her legs. Edna spends all her time sitting in a green armchair. She does not leave this armchair even at night, despite having been advised to elevate her legs and spend the night in bed in order to improve and speed the healing of the ulcers. I built my picture of my patient: an old, very stubborn and recalcitrant lady.

It is human nature to believe that we have good insight as to what we are, but life events let us realise this is only our projection of ourselves and can be completely different from the reality. Before I met Edna I had believed I was nonjudgmental and not a prejudiced person. What struck me about this incident was how easy it could be to label the patient and believe in the infallibility of one's judgment. I had 2 years' experience of working with elderly people and, unfortunately, I developed on the back of this the image of myself as a very good carer. As it turned out that's all it was: just an image. This incident helped me to understand how much I still have to learn to become an effective healthcare professional. After the second or third visit my opinion about Edna was fully formed. I have to admit her attitude irritated me. I could not understand why she could not do what she was asked to do, why she could not do what was going to be beneficial both for her legs and for her general wellbeing, why she did not want to listen to my practice teacher and the good advice she was giving her.

In addition, I could not understand why my practice teacher was so patient with Edna and did not try to assert her view on the role of body positioning to recovery. I was wondering what made my practice teacher was so tolerant and understanding whilst caring for such a difficult and uncooperative individual. I observed Edna for more than a month and my impatience with Edna's behaviour grew inside me. Finally, I let myself share my opinion about Edna with my practice teacher – she did not comment on it, she just told me the secret of Edna's green armchair: it had been her husband's favourite chair. At that very moment my brain 'exploded', it was like a 'storm' of feelings entering my head: I felt so guilty and ashamed of my previous opinions about Edna.

I felt overwhelming guilt that I could be such a cold-hearted person. I could not believe I had been so blind and unwilling to get to know Edna first and thus understand her behaviour. At that very moment I saw for the first time the real and full picture of the patient: a vulnerable, scared, lonely old lady clinging to the vestiges of her husband. I asked myself what I had missed at the beginning of my relationship with Edna and realised that I had not asked myself a few simple questions: why was she like that? Why did she not listen to the nurse? What lay beneath her behaviour? What did I really know about her as a person? Knowing the answers to these questions would not tell me exactly what to do, to try to understand what it was like stand in her shoes.

McCormack (2003: 204) says that the desires, wishes and needs of an older person can be best understood by having a picture of the person's life as a whole; a biography. I had not

(continued)

(continued)

taken the trouble to get to know Edna and I could not therefore see the whole picture of her; only a fragment. Seeing this fragment – an old lady in a chair – had given me false ideas and I had built a false theory on them: Edna was a stubborn patient. I did not see the little girl she had been many years ago, then beautiful young woman. I did not see the happily married woman, with a loving husband and children. I did not see her grief when her daughter passed away from cancer, her everyday longing after her sons, now living far away only visiting from time to time, nor did I see the death of her beloved husband just six months earlier. I did not see her loneliness and her awareness that she was close to the end of her life. Seeing all of this it was suddenly easy to understand why she wanted to sit on the green armchair all the time – it was like a bridge connecting her with her husband and happier times. My involvement with Edna has made me think about the position of the student nurse and my future career as a registered nurse, making me reflect on so many elements which go into the making of good nursing care. It has made me realise the real meaning and importance of holistic care. Holistic nursing care takes into account all aspects of the patient – body, mind and spirit. This underpins all therapeutic nursing interventions (Peate, 2006). My mistake lay in not seeing the person in the patient – it was just another case: venous ulcers which had to be healed. I did not see the individual with all her beliefs, values and life experience, which I should know and respect. Whilst the scientific facts and technical competence are as important as the adoption of a more holistic approach (McCormack, 2003: 203), my vision of this patient ignored the mind and spirit of Edna. I had wanted to care for the patient's body alone.

Now I realise the significance of concordance, 'a partnership of equals on which care plan is negotiated' (McKinnon, 2011: 69). Regrettably, I had represented the concept of compliance – the nurse as an expert. There had been no place for Edna as a partner for me. I had not tried to understand her viewpoint but had wanted to decide what was good for her. The person – centeredness, the mindset in which the interpretations and concerns of the person have primacy in care and fuel care planning (McKinnon, 2011: 70) had been excluded. This person – centeredness can be facilitated when three important factors are considered: the patient's values, the nurse's values and expertise, and the context of care (McCormack, 2003: 205). Patients in advanced age in particular are vulnerable to not being treated as equal partners, and their autonomy, wishes, and independence are overridden in the name of so-called wellbeing. I realised it was so easy to talk at an older person instead of effectively communicating with them. Effective communication requires the emotional involvement of both sides: the patient and the nurse. Older patients, especially, need to see genuine interest not only in their health problems but also in their values, beliefs and their lives in general, in order for them to be active and cooperative in their care.

'And now here is my secret, a very simple secret; it is only with the heart that one can see rightly, what is essential is invisible to the eye' (Saint-Exupery, 2000: 16).

Nurses should be the artists of caring. Each nurse–patient relationship is like a piece of art in the hands of the nurse – to make this piece of art perfect the nurse has to use all possible talents – one of the most important of which is being able to use the heart to see what is invisible for the eyes.

In many ways the incident has a transforming effect on Pilarska: a process we will discuss later in Chapter 6. There is room for another mental footnote here. Pilarska's experience is potent but it is also negative. Informed thinking in practice emerges from an episode in which the student learns from a series of mistaken assumptions and judgements. While this is entirely legitimate as argued earlier in this chapter it does not represent the sole nature of significant events. Such events can highlight good practice which can be shared with others as illustrated in the experience of Richard Simpson (Box 4.4).

Box 4.4   A skill for practice

By Richard Simpson, first year nursing student

Just a few weeks into my first clinical placement I was inexperienced in working with insulin. But I could never have known that the patient I was about to visit that day, a diabetic, would help me realise something about myself that stretched far beyond the management of diabetes. My practice teacher had warned me that Sam (a pseudonym used in line with NMC code (2015)) suffered from mood swings so I was careful to introduce myself, engage in conversation and take extra time to ensure I had obtained informed consent from him before I drew up the insulin.

Then it happened. Sam lashed out swinging a right hook in my direction that would have served any heavyweight boxer well. To this day I have no idea how he missed me (although he could have only missed me by a few centimetres) or how I managed to dodge his fist. But after I did I backed off and before my practice teacher could intervene I had spoken to him in a soft tone asking him to 'take it easy' and reassuring him that I realised he didn't know me but that I wasn't going to hurt him. I let Sam know that I understood he was unsettled by a 'new face'. My practice teacher moved to intervene again but as quickly as his temper had flared up Sam appeared to calm down. The insulin was administered and we left.

In the car we discussed what had happened and my practice teacher commended me for how well I had handled the incident. I responded by saying how much I had surprised myself but then I realised that none of this was new to me. I had grown up with a father who was a recovered alcoholic who in sudden fits of rage or moments of sheer awkwardness and bloody mindedness frequently took his temper out on my mother and me. Such experiences are common among the children and partners of alcoholics and those with alcohol problems (Velleman, Copello and Maslin, 1998). For some years, no one day was the same and what seemed a sensible approach to life at home at one point would be quite impractical on another occasion. My father was someone who seemed at times to want to pick a quarrel for the sheer hell of it. So I learned through bitter experience how to change my tone of voice, body language and to alter how much or how little I said in response. Often my response was simply 'Okay Dad'. At other times the best strategy was to keep my mouth shut and leave quickly if I could. I don't doubt for a moment that I bear some mental and emotional

(continued)

(continued)

scars from my childhood. On the other hand, it seems I have not walked away from those experiences empty handed.

Many children who grow up in emotionally abusive environments prove resilient, developing ways of coping and emerging with life skills they might not otherwise have had. Such resilience can be inherited but also nurtured through support from within and without the family unit (Goldstein and Brooks, 2006). This would seem to have proved true for me. My behaviour in response to Sam has been identified by Linsley (2006) as part of a larger appropriate response to aggression. Linsley stresses the importance of adopting and maintaining a calm demeanour together with interpreting and acknowledging the concerns of the aggressive person. This approach works to stem what Linsley calls the 'escalation phase' (49). Such deescalating person centred behaviour contrasts with an authoritarian approach which is likely to provoke the aggressor to even further aggression and violence.

Since my encounter with Sam I have called upon this 'deescalating' skill a number of times with patients and relatives who express their anger and aggression towards me. I understand that behaviour does not define a person. A person's concerns define a person and are projected in behaviour which may misrepresent their intentions. My father 's behaviour had many fears, regrets and insecurities at its roots and my relationship with him is the better for accepting this. In the same way nursing care which looks beyond behaviour and is shaped around a patient's concerns is essential. There is also another reason why I feel a sense of confidence and pride in this area of practice. Nelms and Lane (1999) have argued that within any group of new recruits to nursing there are mature individuals who have readily developed skills and abilities and are looking for a profession in which to practise them. As a young man only months out of my teens I had never thought of myself as such a person. However, the incident with Sam has helped me see that I have turned around a sad time in my life by using a skill for practice developed from life experience to help others.

Simpson's experience presents an interesting contrast with that of Pilarksa. Pilarska's account reveals to her what was already known to others and related this to person centred theory. In Pilarska's case the 'knowing what' was owned before the 'knowing how'. Simpson's story revealed the unconscious knowing state of his ability up until it was behaviourally experienced in a clinical context. In Simpson's case the 'knowing how' was owned before the 'knowing what'. This truly critical or pivotal incident opened up awareness of personal strengths he brought to nursing and the evidence base to support those strengths meriting the sharing of the narrative with others. An appraisal of Simpson's experience leads us to reevaluate our own family origins and how they may influence our practice for good. As discussed in Chapter 1, positive self-awareness is fuelled through the realisation of skills we may have underestimated or failed to appreciate.

A comparison of Pilarska's narrative with that of Simpson's also serves to once again discharge an old fashioned notion that practice is only about learning how to apply knowledge. Practice also produces knowledge of its own by affirming, challenging or questioning established theory. Notice

Table 4.1 Identifying and harnessing critical incidents

You have experienced a critical incident if an event has:

- had a profound positive or negative effect on you;
- proved emotionally demanding;
- been instrumental in making a difference to something or someone;
- helped you make a connection between two issues which had previously seemed unrelated;
- caused you to think deeply about some aspect of life.

Potential sources of critical incidents

• Surprises	• Epiphanies	• Crises
• Problems	• Dilemmas	• Victories
• Difficulties	• Near misses	• Disasters
• Challenges	• Changes of heart and mind	

Feelings you might experience

Confident	Determined	Elated	Shocked
Proud	Frustrated	Surprised	Awed
Bewildered	Helpless	Powerless	Satisfied
Valued	Respected	Frightened	Angry
Amazed	Uncertain	Uneasy	Threatened
Excited	Relieved	Isolated	Empowered

Incident analysis

Begin writing a personal account of what happened. Be sure to include:

- the context (time, place, location and what was going on);
- your thoughts, emotions, meanings and concerns and at the time of the incident and those which you harbour now if they are different;
- the underpinning issues worthy of discussion.

Take a break to explore through further reading the evidence (research, theories or policies) to support different perspectives on the incident:

- Weave the evidence into your discussion.
- Cite and list your references.
- Describe how this informs your practice.
- State why the outcome of your analysis is worth sharing.

too how both Pilarska and Simpson derive greater learning from their experience through exploration of the research and theory pertaining to their incidents.

The ability of learners to perceive contextual meaning in experience relevant to their own purposes, compare meanings across contexts and behave creatively on the basis of this explains the worth of critical incidents. Table 4.1 might help you think about ways to identify critical incidents in your life and harness them for good in your practice.

Conclusion

A critical incident (sometimes called a significant event) is a happening which is deemed significant by the person who experiences it in that they open a window of opportunity for critical evaluation of some aspect of life. It is set apart from the rest of reflective activity in that no search for meaning is required. It is a 'lightbulb moment' in which meaning is suddenly made apparent to the learner. Thinking of this kind is characterised by tangential and intuitive thought which appreciates the unexpected and unpredictable as having learning potential. The neural dynamics of memory and emotion explain the accelerated nature of learning arising from critical incidents together with the diverse vault of experiences which may contribute to this. The event can be positive or negative and special care needs to be taken to value the former as much as the latter. Our personal makeup and the culture in which we work and live may cause us to concentrate on negative experiences. While negative events have value we need to also realise that as adults with rich diverse experience in life we have the power to be resourceful and innovative. Positive experiences have value too.

5 Towards critical reflection

> ## Box 5.1   Main points: Chapter 5
>
> - Critical reflection questions the assumptions and premises upon which our interpretation of an experience is based at social, cultural, political, psychological and ethical levels. Doing so creates a superior form of meaning making.
> - The meaning of experiences contained within narratives needs to be extracted, decoded, and uncloaked in order to inform practice life.
> - Critical reflection is more accurately represented as a spiral rather than a cycle.
> - Models of critical reflection assist some learners to focus on a range of themes concealed within an experience. They are an optional means rather than a essential end in themselves.

Introduction

This is the chapter which takes us from a *descriptive* to an *analytical* level. This means that while in Chapter 2 we tried to demonstrate knowledge and skill in action within our practice, in this chapter we need to determine the measure of different skills and knowledge required of a care situation. In Chapter 2 we sought to understand the evidence base underpinning our practice but in this chapter we seek to assimilate sets of evidence or theoretical frameworks to inform our practice. In Chapters 1 and 2 we sought greater self-awareness but in this chapter we conduct self-appraisal in the light of research and theory; we ask ourselves how we and our practice have to change in view of what we have learned.

Many learners anticipate that this form of reflecton will be more difficult. However, mature learners often feel more at home thinking at this level. It is as if they recognise in academic form skills they have been using everyday in life.

Moving towards critical reflection

If reflection is how we turn experience into learning, critical reflection is how we analyse, refine and add depth and breadth to learning from that experience.

For Fook (2010: 50) critical reflection is 'the ability to understand the social dimensions and political functions of experience and meaning making and the ability to apply this understanding in working in social contexts'.

In a court of law or other judicial forum any testimony provided by a witness as evidence is subjected to scrutiny by the advocate for the other side. The aim of cross examination is to discredit the story's evidence value by exposing assumption and prejudice which may have warped the interpretation. The environmental conditions in which interpretation shaped judgement may also be brought into question. For example the amount of available daylight and the density of a crowd both affect the ability of a person to view what is happening and report on it accurately. Surrounding distractions such as noise, multiple conversations and the speed with which events take place may create distraction limiting the ability to accurately recall the detail and order of what takes place. Witnesses are also required to consider the testimony of other witnesses whose evidence may conflict with theirs and explain the reason for the difference. Most crucially for the professional use of critical reflection is the role of external evidence. Expert witnesses in court such as pathologists, psychologists, medical doctors, social workers and indeed nurses will produce scientific and practice evidence to support the feasibility of their particular perspective. However, cross examiners will attempt to contest such evidence or the witness's interpretation of it by introducing alternative interpretations and explanations. The court must then consider the meaning of the evidence for the case before it.

In reflection we profess to use our experience as evidence of learning so we must subject this evidence to a similar level of scrutiny. We become our own cross examiner. We revisit our account repeatedly and different perspectives on our assumptions. Instead of simply finding published evidence to support our preordained view we openly enquire into the 'best' evidence by comparing research findings relating to our experience. This is done through exploring expert guidance but also through a search of the literature for original research papers. Finally we must consider the meaning of our learning for our practice and our personal outlook on life.

The notion held by many nurses that critical reflection has always been practised in nursing under a range of different terms (Reid, 1993) is a misinformed one at odds with the evidence. Bullying and harrassment would not be endemic in healthcare if nurses were regularly reflecting ethically on their practice attitudes (RCN, 2005; Francis, 2013), nor would racial discrimination be the regular experience of many nurses at the hands of their peers and managers (Giddings, 2005). The nursing world would be a much better place if we were all as skilled in critical self-appraisal and questioning of the status quo as we like to think we are.

To learn the principles and skills of critical reflection we begin by revisiting the process of reflection in greater depth than that considered in Chapter 2. Kolb's cycle (1988) on which the cycle in Figure 2.1 in Chapter 2 is based provides an opportunity to do this and for ease of understanding the structure will be referred to as if it were the face of a clock (Figure 5.1). Each quandrant of Kolb's cycle involves a different style of thinking and learning and most practitioners will find some more easily to engage with than others.

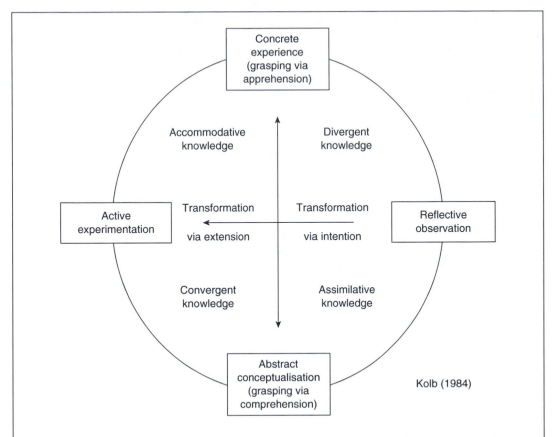

Kolb's cycle of reflection is the framework upon which Gibb's Cycle of Reflection is based. At '12 o'clock' the **concrete experience** represents the story and the first quadrant relates to the trawl of the diverse recalled detail or divergent knowledge present in the story. Revisiting this results in a clearer understanding of the account or **reflective observation** at '3 o'clock'. The second quadrant extending from '3 o'clock' to '6 o'clock' is concerned with realising the salient points in the account worthy of further consideration or assimilative knowledge. At '6 o'clock' a set of isolated principles from the account have been assimilated. This is **abstract conceptualisation.** The third quadrant between '6 o'clock' and '9 o'clock' involves the sifting of the principles of the story together with relevant existing evidence to produce a set of learning which is ready to be transferred to other contexts. This is convergent knowledge. This heralds the beginning of **active experimentation** and the fourth quadrant located between '9 o'clock' and '12 o'clock'. The fourth quadrant concerns the application of the new learning in practical life. This is called accommodative knowledge because the learner literally accommodates or makes room for new knowledge in his way of living and working. Within the cycle the vertical axis stretching from '12 o'clock' and '6 o'clock' represents the comprehension process by which the learner moves from merely apprehending or perceiving an experience to fully understanding it. The horizontal axis stretching from '3 o'clock' to '9 o'clock' represents the transformation process in which the learner moved from owning a detailed knowledge of an experience to being able to apply learning from it. The transformation begins 'via intention' in that the learner sees purpose in the experience and is able to 'extend' this to action which demonstrates application of the learning.

Figure 5.1 Kolb's cycle

Divergent knowing and reflective observation

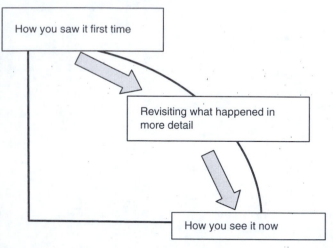

Figure 5.2 Divergent knowing

At '12 o'clock' apprehension of an experience produces divergent knowledge which can be assimilated through reflective observation by '3 o'clock'. We usually remember events in an initially disjointed way. Parts of the story may appear clear while others are vague. The knowledge from the story is in a *divergent* state. Essentially this quandrant is concerned with sifting through and making sense of a story or experience. This may include:

- Reliving the experience several times in our minds.
- Establishing a chronological order.
- Clarifying all the 'players' in the story including who said what.
- Remembering additional detail in the shape of the vocal tone, attitude, facial expression and body language of those involved including ourselves.
- Attempting to ascertain the motives and values of those involved including yourself.

Individuals who excel in this part of the learning cycle have a good imagination and are able to consider a situation from a variety of perspectives. Evidence suggests that women have the advantage over men in this part of the reflective process. The corpus callosum which connects both hemispheres is more bulbous and contains more axons and dendrites in women. Women also have wider peripheral vision than men. This shows that women are able to conduct a broader assessment of a situation in which human behaviour is key; utilising more brain centres simultaneously (Solms and Turnbull, 2002; Baron-Cohen, 2003) However, everyone can improve their reflective observation by reliving the experience in their minds and if possible discussing this with others.

Assimilative knowing and abstract conceptualisation

Assimilative knowing makes it possible for us to *assimilate, embrace or grasp and take in* the clearer version of our story which presents at '3 o'clock'. Assimilative knowledge takes us from

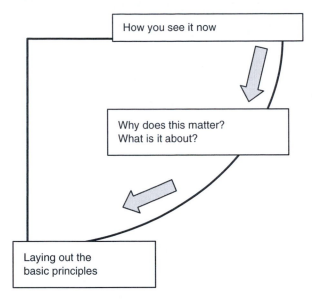

Figure 5.3 Assimilative knowing

reflective observation to abstract conceptualisation. By '6 o'clock', the point of abstract conceptualisation, we are able to understand why the story is important to us and extract the principles and concepts underpinning the story which can be transferred to other settings at other times. This is comprehension. We abstractly conceptualise everyday of our lives. This is most often practised with our children as we explain at pedestrian pace the 'lessons' that they should learn from something that they have done. In the same way at the stage of abstract conceptualistion we should possess a set of knowledge and principles which are new to us which we believe are valuable for our future practice. The role of active listening in history taking, the importance of patient confidentiality, asepsis in wound care, handwashing in the control of antimicrobial resistance and the benefits of work life balance in nursing are all examples from an infinitely long list of abstract concepts. So assimilative knowing is about:

- Understanding why the story matters to us.
- Determining the principles underpinning the story.

An assimilative thinker is naturally reflective and able to grasp theory underpinning an experience. We can develop sound assimilative skills by repeatedly exploring our emotions relating to an experience and the reason for these emotions. This will help us to explore why the experience matters to us and this in turn will expose the principles at work in the story (Illeris, 2007).

Convergent knowing

Convergent knowing occurs between abstract conceptualisation and active experimentation at '9 o'clock'. Convergent knowing will begin by comparing the principles deduced from the internal evidence of our experience with the messages from external evidence in research, theory and policy. At this point there is a need to revisit and remember some fundamental principles of reflection:

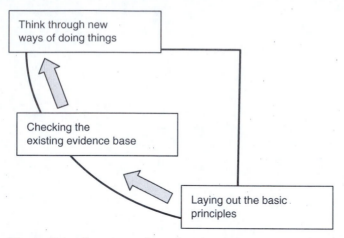

Figure 5.4 Convergent knowing

- Reflection is not all about exposing our failings. It is also about endorsing good practice. So at the endpoint of our reflection we may have reason to be proud of our practice as much as to criticise it.
- Reflection informs practice but it is also informed by practice.
- Extant literature may have a bearing on our learning but our experience in practice may also pose questions for further research. Questions from 'real life' are what feed further research and force changes to policy.

After this the learner should consider how this new learning can be practically applied. This would include a consideration of the barriers to change and how these barriers can be negotiated. If we have cause to share positive findings we still need to decide the best way of doing this; for example publication, discussing at a team meeting, designing a new template of standards, writing a proposal for management or a combination of all of these. Convergent knowing is:

- A 'narrowing down' or reduction process. Our reflections '*converge*' on the usefulness of our experience.
- Thinking about new ways of working and doing things in the light of our reflection.

A person with a convergent learning style is an expert problem solver because they are able to swifty apply new knowledge and skills. Convergent learners do not become entrenched in the problem. Instead they move quickly toward finding a solution. A comparison of the learners conclusions with the recommendations of external research and policy will assist everyone to improve their convergent knowing.

Accommodative knowing

In the last quadrant of Kolb's cycle the learner literally 'makes room for' or accomodates new learning in his life.

Accomodative learning begins with active experimentation or learning by doing and ends with the synthesis of new knowledge in a new setting. Accommodative thinkers are creative and intuitive, able to advance toward critical challenging levels of reflection without any precursor stages. Accommodative

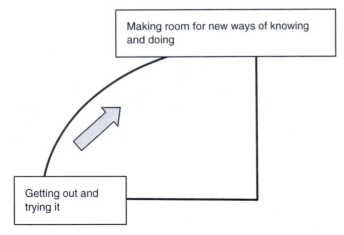

Figure 5.5   Accommodative knowing

thinkers are able to challenge taken for granted meanings and assumptions. They are able to spiral upwards through a range of levels of ethical, personal, cultural and sociopolitical knowing reshaping their approaches and sometimes themselves as a result. So accomodative knowing is about:

- Accommodating or *'making room for'* new knowledge arising from reflection.
- Thinking about who and what might present as barriers to your new ways of working and how these might be negotiated.
- Having the courage to apply new knowledge.

If we accept that life learning comes from interaction with our world then we must also accept that our thinking will be heavily influenced by what is deemed acceptable, appropriate, fair, right and reasonable by individuals and institutions around us some of whose motives may be highly questionable. Equally our own assumptions and motives may warrant closer examination in the light of evidence. How is this done?

Oleson (1989: 21) has argued that 'reality is not immediately apparent'. The value of this is found in the basis for our interpretations. There are two types of meaning making. Meaning Schemes are constructed after our learned expectations of what we see, the sequences of events and the cause and effect relationships taken from our limited experience. The view from our front door when it is opened, food satisfying hunger and water satisfying thirst are all examples of meaning schemes. These schemes become implicit rules for interpretation. Meaning perspectives are higher order argument sets than that of meaning schemes. Meaning perspectives consist of beliefs, values and theories which are applied in our life interpretations (Kitchenham, 2008). For example, the idea that hard work automatically leads to success and prosperity is born of such a perspective. Critical reflection is concerned with challenging the assumptions at work within these taken for granted meaning schemes and perspectives which punctuate our lives. These taken for granted meanings require deconstructing or 'picking apart'. Deconstruction involves several tasks:

1. **Extraction** is necessary in that meaning is embedded in the fabric of memory footage and narrative; the story together with the concern it arouses, the issues it produces and the principles it highlights.

2. **Decoding** is necessary because language and the interstices of language may contain subtle messages quite different from those which are perceived prima facie. 'Nurse team reprofiling' may be presented by health service managers as an innovative response to changing need. However, if such reprofiling saves money by reducing the level of expertise in the team rather than varying the type of expertise then the terms of reference for the whole exercise may be disingenuous. Life would be much easier if everyone wore their prejudices 'on their sleeves' exposed for everyone to see as is the case with many extremist political and religious zealots. Instead in the case of many individuals, communities, groups and organisations, cleverly crafted language and social excuses may code for discrimination, bigotry and hatred.

3. **Uncloaking** is distinct from decoding in that it seeks to uncover meaning, aims, values, motives and messages that are deliberately hidden as opposed to those which are simply initially unperceived. For example government and organisation policy documents are often presented in an instructional way which does not appear to permit the reader a choice or any consideration of the underpinning assumptions and values which may be misguided.

4. **Informing** is the point of application in critical reflection; the stage at which we answer the question 'What does this mean for me and my practice?'. Friere (2005) argued that even if critical reflection does not provide the means to address new perspectives on situations, the reflective practitioner still exists closer to reality than before and is therefore better informed. Friere called this 'conscienzation'. An informed position even in the absence of any apparent solution or option for change still places the nurse in a more powerful position; enabled to practise decisions, explain deficits and argue for change. An informed position also helps one realise one's true worth in an environment where one is undervalued.

When we deconstruct our experiences we begin to inform our practice at a critical level. Reflection has been compared to an onion; composed of many 'layers of meaning' (Korthagen and Vasolos, 2005). Just like an onion the more we peel the more there is to peel. The more we reflect on the 'layers' of an experience the more there is to reflect upon. The knowledge waiting to be discovered in any experience is deceptively complex. Considering a number of themes will prove helpful.

Social themes

Society is constructed. It does not grow out of some universal consensus but is structured in a way which favours the most powerful. A matrix of myths and legends has been fabricated to help sustain the status quo by implying that existing systems stand in their place through merit rather than privilege. In reality, inheritance, gender, ethnicity, the family and house of one's birth, education pathways and the health and wellbeing of one's parents all forge one's place in society far more than any measure of merit. It is true that in the democratic world individuals and pressure groups lobby successfully for change which delivers justice on behalf of the disadvantaged. However, the existence of such societal tension only serves to illustrate the unequal balance of power which characterises human affairs past and present. From free education and healthcare to universal suffrage and racial equality the rights which people possess have always been won following long and bitter struggles and never out of some sense of beneficent duty on the part of those holding power. Responsibility and blame is placed with victims of inequality and disadvantage to disguise deficits in the system and absolve

the powerful (Haramlambos and Holborn, 2013). Research has shown that a plurality of negative health and social behaviours issue from the frustration, diminished choice and learned helplessness that partners poverty and disadvantage (Graham and Power, 2005; Vansteenkiste and Ryan, 2013).

Power imbalance is a fault running through contemporary society characterising relationships between politicians and the electorate, teachers and students, employers and employees, women and men and nurses and their patients. The part played by power in relationships can be often exposed using a reversal technique recommended by the social research theorists, Strauss and Corbin (1990). The technique involves reversing the roles of the individuals involved in a situation to see if the outcome is correspondingly changed. Such a reversal approach involving men and women, medicine and nursing, adults and children, Caucasian and non-Caucasian ethnic groups to name but a few can be very revealing.

Reflecting on social themes contained within an experience can lift veils of prejudice among nurses toward the most vulnerable in our society including smokers, drug addicts, homeless people and people with suicidal behaviour, older people and children. Socially aware practice can not only provide more effective and appropriate care but work towards empowering individuals and groups for greater participation in society (Lavarack, 2009).

Box 5.2   Examples of critical questioning

- What does government policy say about this and what effect does this have?
- What research exists to support one side or the other in the issue(s) that arose?
- How relevant is the gender, ethnicity and culture of the people involved?
- What does this reveal about how older people are sometimes viewed in western contemporary society?
- What does this experience tell me about a person's spiritual needs?
- What does this experience tell me about the duty of the nurse to care for patients and society and is there conflict between the two?

Cultural themes

Every community from a professional team to a city or a nation has a culture. Culture is a toolkit for understanding and managing one's world (Bruner, 1999). Meaning is gradually attributed by a young child to a range of semiotics including mimicry, signs, symbols, vocal, facial and body expression. The intrigued child is able to tease and test out the meaning through participation in social behaviour. In turn social behaviour including speech develops further on the basis of what is gleaned, interpreted and internalised from the social domain. Dialects and dialogue both reflect local and global social and cultural mores of the time period in which they take place. This is audible in the vernacular and adolescent slang of one decade and location in comparison to others. Moreover, the most articulate speech is incomplete without complementary semiotics to lend illustration, emphasis, reinforcement, and additional sense to the spoken word. Words are delivered with meaning and in context through use of gestures, facial expressions, signs and symbols (Robbins, 2001).

Culture is a socially established way of knowing, understanding, doing, expressing and communicating which identifies one community and era from another. It is a lens through which we see our world providing the boundaries of what is right and acceptable and what is to be rejected as unacceptable. In any human interaction a failure to acknowledge culture will inevitably lead to many misinterpretations and misunderstandings (Habermas, 1970).

Culture evolves over time under the influence of its membership but because of the limited lifespan of birth cohort members, it exerts a far greater influence on them than the other way around. Organisations and working teams also have a culture which influences the behaviour of its members. Such work cultures can be characterised by work life balance, listening management, mutual respect and recognition, reward for hard work and promotion of wellbeing. Alternatively, a place of work can feature draconian management, bullying and harrassment, workloads that are not sustainable and be toxic to the wellbeing of those who are employed there (Francis, 2013).

Culture is our nurse and teacher but it is also our jailor. An individual must consciously and actively draw on critical theory to deconstruct cultural concepts, such is the power of culture over his or her perception of the world and actions (Jarvis, 1992a).

In the Danish language there is no word for 'please'. Graciousness and good manners are captured in the *'way'* one makes a request of others. So when Danish people speak English they have to remember to insert the word 'please' into every request. Even then it may sound as if it has no real meaning to them. To someone unfamiliar with this language characteristic the Danes will almost certainly appear illmannered, rude or even arrogant. The hardened way in which Scottish people sound their consonants together with their more direct method of conversation may appear intimidating to Anglo Saxon people. Alternatively, for Latin people the hardened consonants of the Scots dialect make their spoken English easier to understand. Iraqi war veterans still recall how despite preparation for civilian life in Iraq, American troops often misinterpreted the rapid loud speech and elaborate extended hand and arm gestures of Iraqi civilians as aggression. In nursing practice the different ways in which different national groups express pain has sometimes led to misunderstandings about individual pain thresholds and the need for pain relief. So in the field of linguistics and semiotics alone culture has power to heavily influence and warp interpretation.

Any profession working so closely with humanity as nursing cannot dismiss the implications of culture for person centred care. It must be considered and embraced to inform practice.

Political themes

It is folly to believe that nursing can exist in a politically neutral environment. Everything we do and say in life influences and is influenced by politics (Kitchenham, 2008). All politicians speak passionately about the importance of topics at the forefront of the public mind; education, health, the economy, immigration, defence, the environment and criminal justice are all examples which feature frequently in political rhetoric and debate. So the question arises: as all politicians claim to care about these subjects but often espouse different policies, how can anyone discern which political perspective to own? A closer examination of policy betrays the underpinning assumptions and values on which governments position themselves. The use of social and fiscal research findings can often help us to critique the claims of politicians. For example, the British National Health Service is often implicitly referred to as a burgeoning mushrooming financial burden on the public purse. However, the proportion of gross domestic product reserved for health care in Britain has been among the lowest of the developed nations. The efficacy and appropriateness of universal health care provision is often measured against morbidity figures such as those for cardiovascular disease, cancer, clinical obesity, diabetes, and mental illness. Yet these conditions have their roots in the wider social determinants of health such as poverty, access to cheap fresh produce, work life balance and life chances (Marmot and Wilkinson, 2006). Nurses need to be politically aware, ready and able to make an informed case in order to preserve good practice and safeguard quality patient care.

Ethical themes

Reflecting on ethical themes within experience is about discerning morally right and wrong behaviour. It is important to use an ethical framework together with the code of professional conduct published by the nursing regulatory body of the country within which we practice.

Ethics (originating from the Greek Word 'ethos' meaning character, conduct or custom) and a closely allied word, morals (from the Latin word 'mores' meaning custom or habit) form a branch of philosophy concerned with measuring and determining right and wrong. As nurses, our involvement with large numbers of people negotiating crises brought about by health problems means that we are confronted by large numbers of complex moral predicaments, many of which we have never previously encountered. Frameworks which draw on more diverse philosophical ground than the system which we may personally use are necessary to guide our actions in such situations. Furthermore, patients and their families also use their own moral frameworks as guides for living but on being confronted by mental or physical trauma, coping mechanisms become paralysed or fragmented. Such individuals rely on health care professionals to provide support with their decision making. It is important that practitioners do not permit their own values and beliefs to bias the support they provide. To remain impartial as an ethical helper requires the use of theoretical models (Beauchamp and Childress, 2013). Concepts such as 'prioritising patient autonomy, dignity and confidentiality' 'first doing no harm', 'doing good' and 'acting fairly' will all be concerns of the nurse who is reflecting ethically on her practice. Ethical practice also relates to human qualities of kindness and compassion (Ballot and Campling, 2011). However, in the context of nursing there are often times when ethical principles appear to conflict. For example, patient confidentiality cannot be absolute in issues of suspected child maltreatment and supplying clean needles to drug addicts constitutes beneficence in the prevention of blood borne diseases. Such areas of conflict make ethical reflection essential through use of deontology and other related frameworks. The pace and demands of practice can also cause tension within and between teams and practitioners. Ethical reflection is also important in guiding our behaviour toward colleagues.

Psychological themes

Human behaviour is not the explanation of a person's being. It is a response to their experience of being. The insightful practitioner seeks to understand the underlying causes of a person's behaviour so as to inform their own behaviour as accurately as possible. Considering our experiences in the light of developmental theory and research findings into ontological perspectives supply discernment and empathy in our dealings with diverse patient groups. Our self-knowledge will also be enhanced. For example, reflection on the psychological evidence underpinning human behaviour and ways of working with this behaviour can transform our communication skills (Stickley and Freshwater, 2006), management of challenging and aggressive behaviour (Linsley, 2006) and end of life care (Haley, Larson, Kasl-Godley, Neimeyer and Kwilosz, 2003).

Beyond a cyclical approach to reflection

At this point in the discussion it is important that we realise that while a reflective cycle is useful in helping a novice to learn reflection as a basic process, beyond this it is very limited. In a cycle the majority of the focus is on the story, the context and the self. There is minimal directive to critique the context or think beyond it and there is no encouragement to form links between the experience

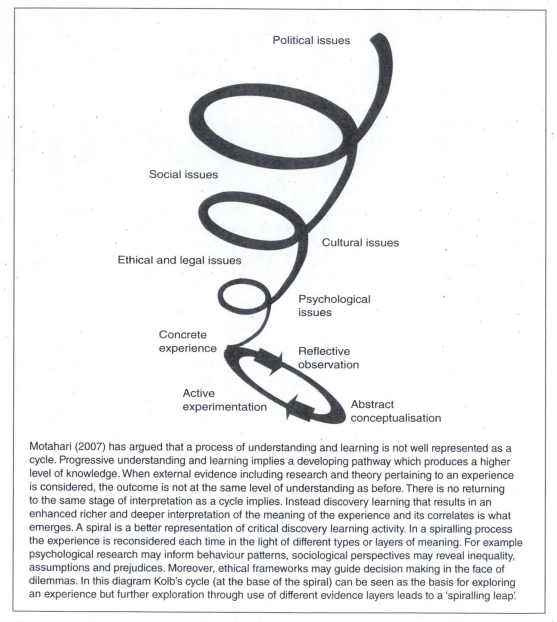

Motahari (2007) has argued that a process of understanding and learning is not well represented as a cycle. Progressive understanding and learning implies a developing pathway which produces a higher level of knowledge. When external evidence including research and theory pertaining to an experience is considered, the outcome is not at the same level of understanding as before. There is no returning to the same stage of interpretation as a cycle implies. Instead discovery learning that results in an enhanced richer and deeper interpretation of the meaning of the experience and its correlates is what emerges. A spiral is a better representation of critical discovery learning activity. In a spiralling process the experience is reconsidered each time in the light of different types or layers of meaning. For example psychological research may inform behaviour patterns, sociological perspectives may reveal inequality, assumptions and prejudices. Moreover, ethical frameworks may guide decision making in the face of dilemmas. In this diagram Kolb's cycle (at the base of the spiral) can be seen as the basis for exploring an experience but further exploration through use of different evidence layers leads to a 'spiralling leap'.

Figure 5.6   The spiral of critical reflection

and the outside world (Talbot, 2012). Motohari's arguments (2007) imply that the reality of critical reflection is more credibly represented as a spiral (Figure 5.6).

The richer the combination of themes explored in an experience the greater number of perspectives that will emerge and greater the learning that will result; deepening our knowledge and broadening our reasoning. Ryan Lusby's critical reflection (Box 5.3) on his relationship with an older patient in his care with dementia shows the value of 'unwrapping' an experience to find different layers of meaning. Lusby pursues several 'themes' in his story which provide clues as to why a patient labelled 'difficult' proved sociable and cooperative in his company. In doing so he finds not one but several possible explanations and concludes that the truth probably lies somewhere within a combination of all of them. Lusby explores cultural and political themes through examination of the evidence for continuity of management of care giving and receiving. He considers the implications of active listening and reminiscing conversation for the wellbeing of vulnerable older people. Lusby also seeks to explain his acceptability through the neuropsychology of memory which informs on the ontology of dementia. Lusby's affirmed confidence in his skills speaks from the page. His humility in the perplexity which triggers his reflection dismisses any notion that his narrative is a self-congratulatory exercise. His work is another example of how reflection should realise excellence in practice as well as learning that arises from negative outcomes and self-criticism.

Box 5.3　The 'difficult' patient that wasn't

By Ryan Lusby, second year nursing student

Morris was a patient that many found to be very difficult to take care of. I was told that he was uncooperative, constantly declined to be washed, always refused his medications (unless it was analgesia), and rejected all oral fluids and any food. But in the week in which he was under my care, I rarely experienced any of these characteristics from Morris. From the first day that I looked after him, I was able to get Morris to eat and take minimal amounts of fluid (still an achievement). It took time but he also agreed to take most, if not all, of his medication. I was even able to have simple conversations with this man whom the majority of the staff on the ward thought to be a challenging individual. I found that all it took was a bit of time, perseverance and improvisation. Prior to helping Morris with his medication, I would ensure that I had his full attention. I engaged him in conversation on a topic completely unrelated to his care; hobbies he used to have, family members close to his heart. It didn't really matter what we talked about. After a few minutes, knowing that I had Morris 'on my side' and in a good mood, I would request that he take his medication for me so that we could help him get better and going home.

As the time that Morris spent on the ward grew longer, so did the quality of the relationship between us. I vividly remember an occasion during one shift, mid-afternoon, when a phlebotomist came onto the ward and into Morris' bay. She was looking for him. What I witnessed next was very similar to what I'd seen take place between Morris and other nurses in the past. For a patient with dementia, I can imagine the world is a rather scary

(continued)

(continued)

place for them to live in; confusion, anxiety, frustration. So for this lady to march up to Morris, check his wristband for identity, and go about setting up her equipment with only a brief explanation and no smile . . . I can only imagine how terrifying this must have been for this poor man.

I was busy with another patient in the same bay as Morris when I witnessed how agitated he was getting; shouting, demanding for this woman to leave him alone. With every passing minute, Morris' was becoming more aggressive, and the phlebotomist's patience was wearing thin. It was at this point that Morris noticed me on the other side of the room and called out. From my recollection, there have been only a handful of moments in my life in which I have felt someone truly, and urgently, needed me. This was one of those moments. The expression on this man's face as I briskly walked over to him was just full of a vast variety of emotions. I saw anxiety, but relief. I noted confusion, but clarity at the same time. Morris looked up at me and asked what was about to happen and why he needed it done. I politely requested that the phlebotomist give me two minutes of privacy with Morris. Slowly, clearly and thoroughly, I explained to him the need for this procedure and enquired as to whether he understood. Still very distressed about this, he was silent for a few seconds, pondering. He turned to me once more and, although I wasn't fully convinced with his answer, he stated that he did understand, and that he would have his blood taken. However, Morris stipulated one condition: he would only have his blood taken if I agreed to stay with him and hold his hand.

I began to ask myself, why and how? Why was I able to get this 'difficult' patient to cooperate? Why did I make Morris feel comfortable and less anxious? How did I get this reaction from this patient?

Continuity is often directly linked with high-standard care. Within continuity there are two distinct dimensions: relationship and management. Relationship continuity relates to the same individual caring for the same patient consistently, thus allowing the development of a therapeutic relationship with the personal security this entails. Management continuity relates to the sharing of information and ensuring a constant and clear approach to the care of all patients (Haggerty, Reid, Freeman, Starfield, Adair and McKendry, 2003: 1219). Relationship continuity is seen as highly appreciated by healthcare professionals and their patients due to the wide range of benefits that comes with it. These include enhanced holistic care, preserved personhood, greater job satisfaction, improved exchange of information, increased likelihood of advice taking, reduced hospital admissions and reduced costs (Freeman and Hughes, 2010).

Continuity is important to me. If I am to work three long days a week, I like to be placed in the same section of a ward, looking after the same patients, to allow me to get to know each and every service user, and so they can also get to know me. I enjoy being able to walk into my delegated part of the ward in the morning, wishing a good morning to those who are already up, and reluctantly awakening the patients that have been lucky enough to sleep through the noise of the night. Some recognise me from the previous days, but yet can't quite remember my name, but that's fine, nothing a simple mind jog won't rectify. Most do remember who I am, and I relish the welcoming smiles and heart-warming gestures.

There is every reason to suppose that continuity was also important to Morris. The fact that I had looked after Morris frequently would have created a better relationship between us, and this could have been something he valued. For patients with dementia, continuity of care is important. Hospitalisation from a nursing home disrupts this continuity for a patient, causing potential problems for the dementia patient (Finucane, Bellantoni and Ouslander, 2013). Having a form of continuity integrated into his care at hospital may have enhanced Morris' experience on the ward.

Effective communication with an individual with dementia is likely to enhance the quality of life of that person, whilst also easing stress on the healthcare professional caring for them (Livingstone, Kelly and Lewis-Holmes, 2014). Helping such patients to reminisce in conversation about hobbies, interests, work history and relationships has been shown to improve communication skill, preserve personal identity and enhance overall mood and wellbeing (Swann, 2013).

However, of all the communication skills, listening is the most difficult to master. If executed efficiently, it has proactive properties in that it can ease anxiety. Listening is not just about hearing, but also involves observing a patient's body language and facial expressions (McKinnon, 2011).

I have gradually developed my interpersonal skills during my studies, and I am able to adapt my manner appropriately to each individual that I care for. I have quickly learned that listening and understanding what your patient wants and needs is a vital aspect of nursing. For me the individual in question knows the most about their needs, so the best thing to do is *listen*. What are they telling you? Act upon this. Are they in pain? Rectify that.

Morris may have valued this in me. His anxiety was of great concern to me and I ensured I took the time to listen to him and work to ease any worries he had. When someone is expressing their feelings and concerns it is not enough to just listen. It is important to *show* them that you are listening too. I have learned that giving facial feedback is an effective way of doing this. Matching the person's body language also shows them you are listening but also makes it easier to have empathy and can create greater understanding (McKinnon, 2011). Listening and empathic patterns of behaviour coupled with caring actions are what form trust: the foundation for care planning and coordination which is acceptable and creates minimum anxiety (Pask, 1995). Morris may have taken note of the effort I made to listen to his worries, something he might have been craving since being admitted to the ward. The cooperation I received from Morris could have been because of this.

Suffering from dementia, Morris experienced bouts of agitation and confusion. His confusion was not constant, but frequent. Never the less patients like Morris are still able to recall the distant past. It is generally short-term memory that is most affected. Patients will

(continued)

(continued)

commonly have difficulty remembering what happened minutes, hours, or days ago, but may be able to recall, sometimes in great detail, moments in life when they were younger. This is because after context tied episodic memory has fragmented, personal semantic memory functions independently (Joubert, Mauries, Barbeau, Ceccaldi, and Poncet, 2004). It is therefore possible that I reminded Morris of a family member or old friend from his youth, explaining why he reacted to me in such a unique way.

All patients are different in some way or another. Some will be easy to care for, some, not so much. This experience with Morris has taught me to not be daunted by a 'difficult' patient. If I use everything I have been taught I know I can have a positive impact on someone's care. The reaction I received from Morris has affirmed in me the importance of delivering as high a standard of nursing practice as possible at all times, regardless of the patient.

Although I was warned that Morris would be a 'handful' to care for, I found that it was quite the opposite. Nursing Morris turned out to be an experience that I will never forget, for very positive reasons. I feel privileged to have been responsible for his care and to have been part of his care experience.

Models of critical reflection

Any model or framework is a concept map which demonstrates to the learner the relationships between essential parts of praxis to enhance professional movement. A model bids to accurately represent efficient and effective thinking in the mind of the user. It follows from this that a framework that is ideal for everyone in every situation will prove elusive. The nature of the experience will often dictate the type of reflection that is required. Nursing academia has become accustomed to requiring the use of a model by a learner in a piece of reflection. However, as it is adherence to principles rather than a particular thinking pathway that is key here; the mere use of a model is by itself unlikely to guarantee a good standard of critical reflection. A model to guide critical reflection is a matter for personal choice but as a rule of thumb any such framework should sit neatly across three functions:

1. Provide sufficient structure to 'signpost' thinking in a way that will 'milk' an experience for the maximum amount of learning that it can supply.
2. Provide sufficient freedom so that the learner is not pushed along an 'over prescribed' route punctuated with over precise signposts that serve to block exploration of other valuable lines of thought.
3. Enable a critique of taken for granted meanings and habitual thinking which prevail within an experience.

One such model among many is Barbara Carper's *Fundamental Patterns of Knowing in Nursing* (1978) (Box 5.4). The model does not signpost a pathway of reflection but instead provides cues which together are intended to encompass all the constituents of knowing in nursing. There is some overlap in meaning represented by the four headings within the model and so the user may choose to use these headings or discard them in favour of a more integrated approach. If the latter approach is preferred, then using the language of the model will help maintain a connection between the text and the framework's values.

Box 5.4   Carper's patterns of knowing in nursing

As in the case of many models of critical reflection, Barbara Carper lays emphasis, not in direction of the learning process but in the layers of learning hidden in an experience. Direction of learning process is left to the learner. The dividing lines between each domain are not rigid but involve considerable overlap. For example an examination of evidence is important in every domain and ethical considerations will inevitably involve self-awareness.

Empirical

When practice is populated with many repetitive tasks, ways of working can easily be fashioned after how things have been done in the past or what appears to be right at the time. In the empirical domain, the learner is encouraged to question the evidence for what he assumes; his beliefs, values and what he *thinks* he knows. In any professional community of practice skills and knowledge are essentially handed down from masters to apprentices (Wenger, 1999; Polanyi, 1999). This important process carries risk in that practice removed from a credible evidence base risks being steeped in personal opinion and outdated, discredited values. Time honoured tradition and ritualistic ways of working will take precedence over science informing artful practice. Consequently practice may become inappropriate, ineffective, unethical and even dangerous. Empirical patterns of knowing are concerned with the search for evidence in the extant literature to validate, refute or clarify the issues and principles that issue from an experience in practice. The following questions are all pertinent:

- What meaning does the evidence have for the experience?
- What bearing does this evidence have on taken for granted assumptions and values?
- What questions are raised by the evidence which require further exploration?
- How is best practice forged from the evidence?

Empirical knowing assists the reflective practitioner to think critically by driving a comparison between actual practice and the evidence (research, theory and policy) pertaining to that practice.

Aesthetic

As a footballer crosses the field with the ball at his feet he will use a range of skills; some simultaneously and others in a pre-programmed order to reach the most appropriate point at

(continued)

(continued)

which he should attempt to score or pass the ball effectively to a team member. It is highly unlikely that in these crucial moments he will be conscious of the way he uses certain major muscle groups in his feet, limbs and torso to guide the ball with precision. Nor will he give any thought to his eye foot coordination or how in turn this is coordinated with his direction and speed of movement together with his awareness of other players' shifting positions. An array of sport science evidence will underpin his training and preparation but in the moment of execution this will be the last thing on his mind. The very nature of the art of his game means that a complex range of skills must be unified in a modulated polished performance. In a similar way the everyday nature of nursing practice means that the complex combination of skills used in response to client need may go unrealised and unappreciated (Schon, 1987). The aesthetic layer holds the essence of the 'artistry' in practice. It is concerned with the way the parts of practice relate to the whole and the way in which the whole is greater than the sum of its parts. In this domain the nurse is seen as an artist with a palate from which she selects the right colour measure and texture of paint to produce the desired portrait. As a professional practitioner the nurse is equipped with a 'menu' of skills and knowledge: listening skills, pharmacology, patho-physiology, psychology and ethics are examples from an infinitely larger list which make up this professional 'palate'. Different episodes of care call for a different 'mix' of different skills and knowledge areas in different measures. Aesthetics is about exploring the particular 'selection' of skills, qualities and evidence required of a care context and how they are applied appropriately. In the context of partnership working with patients and their families there is a need to recognise that they also contribute to the aesthetics layer as experts in their own lives (Cloutier, Duncan and Bailey, 2007).

Personal

Personal knowing is about self-awareness and use of self as discussed in Chapter 1 but as it informs and is informed by a specific experience. It is about the sort of person we are and our personal development as it pertains to our practice. Awareness of body language, vocal tone, facial expression, attitudes and values (both our own and others) as they are moulded by emotion thought and culture are at the centre of personal knowing (Eckroth-Bucher, 2010). Regardless of our time of life, a new experience may bring more clarity to our self-awareness highlighting strengths previously unrealised and also traits which are undesirable or need further work (Jack and Miller, 2008).

Questions which may arise in the personal domain are:

- Why do I feel uncomfortable in this situation?
- What are the clues to the reasons for this person's behaviour and attitude?
- What does this tell me about the sort of person I am?
- What pointers are there here for my future development?

Both the aesthetic and personal domains are closely connected to 'unwrapping' of intuition and intuitive thought.

Ethical

Ethical knowing is concerned with codes of conduct and moral concepts such as autonomy, non-maleficence, beneficence and justice. Contained within our own personal codes of moral reasoning, many of us harbour ideas about right and wrong which we consider to be absolute in certain situations. Theft, fidelity to one's partner and the sanctity of life are only three examples in which many might take an absolutist stance. In the role of health care practitioner, however, we provide care for many individuals and groups who do not share our views or who may take an absolutist stance on issues we consider to be relative to the context of the situation. Diverse moral codes issue from diverse sources ranging from the teachings of a holy book to a self-constructed framework based on lived experience. Not infrequently individuals allow what is aesthetically pleasing, what intuitively feels right or what seems most practical to guide their actions. Prostitutes, criminals, drug addicts and people with resolute religious or political beliefs will all own frameworks of moral reasoning from which we may wish to distance ourselves or which we may find provocative. Ethical models assist us in acknowledging the right of all patients to receive our care and participate in their own health care plans in a way which fits with their own value system, placing moral relativism as a prerequisite to good practice (Seedhouse, 2008).

However, while ethical concepts and the models they form are guides for behaviour. They do not constitute ethical comportment. Ethical knowing in addition to awareness of good and right behaviour also discerns what is good and right to be (Benner, Tanner and Chesla, 1996).

Michael Lewis-Shermer (Box 5.5) uses Carper's model to critically reflect on an unexpected awkwardness he experiences while removing surgical clips from a patient in the community. He shows that his choice of Carper's model is not academic posturing but a response to his need to relate his personal knowledge to evidence base. Note that while Lewis-Shermer declares his use of Carper at the beginning he changes the order of the headings to suit his own thought process. This is good practice. The model should always fit the experience rather than the other way around. In Lewis-Shermer's case Carper proves valuable. Under the banner of personal knowing, he sources psychology to explain his feelings during the clip removal. This bolsters his self-awareness and he accommodates this knowledge within his continual professional development plan. In the ethical domain Lewis-Shermer identifies non-maleficence as the principle underpinning his decision to refer to his practice teacher the removal of an over granulated surgical clip. His reflection on aesthetics houses an evidence based approach to wound healing within professional judgement. This is the contextualisation of the empirical domain within praxis. Lewis-Shermer's narrative shows how a seemingly brief and insignificant experience can yield a rich 'crop' of learning.

Box 5.5 First time removal of surgical staples in a community setting: a reflective narrative using Carper's patterns of knowing

By Michael Lewis Shermer, third year nursing student

In this reflection I will be using Carper (1987) the Fundamental Patterns of Knowing, because I feel that I want to make a link between my personal knowledge, my moral standing in decision making, and the evidence base for nursing. Carper's model is most suitable for this, because it openly requires me to consider these areas of my practice, and use questions derived from the model to expand on them. I will set out this reflection in a different order to Carper's original model, choosing to discuss personal elements, followed by ethical decisions, empirical evidence, and finally the aesthetics of nursing. I will do this because this will allow me to incorporate all the aspects of this model, while preserving my own thought processes in their natural order.

Surgical staples are specialised clips used in surgery in place of sutures to close surgical site wounds, connect or remove parts of the bowel or lungs. Stapling is much faster than suturing by hand, and is also more accurate and consistent. The removal of staples can be performed in both acute and community settings using a specialised clip remover (Moy et al., 2013).

While on a home visit with my practice teacher, I performed a removal of surgical staples on Roger. Up until this point I had only removed staples in acute settings and the difference in my own confidence while undertaking surprised me. I recognised instantly that I am a lot more confident in acute settings. When removing the staples I noticed one staple that had slightly over granulated, I left this in situ and requested that my practice teacher take over as I felt unable to remove it. This relates to what Carper (1978) calls personal knowing as I had a lack of knowledge and skills to deal with the situation and wanted to learn from my practice teacher's example.

Personal knowing in nursing refers to a distinctively personal type of knowledge constructed of subjective understanding and perspective on personal experience. Personal knowing is a dynamic process and the result of personal reflection and transformation as the individual lives and interacts with their world (Stake, 2000).

I have worked with surgical staples both on hospital wards and in theatres, and in these environments I feel competent performing the removal procedure safely. When I transferred this knowledge to Roger's care in his own home, my confidence decreased. I had discovered that it can be intimidating performing clinical procedures in a quiet intimate setting where the only audience is the patient. The impact of passive spectators on a person's behaviour or skill performance has been defined by Dashiell (1935) as the 'audience effect' under the umbrella term of social facilitation. Dashiell (1935) found that the presence of an audience facilitated

an improvement in the subject's performance and Travis (1925) found that subjects were better at mentally stimulating manual tasks in front of spectators. However, in my own situation I experienced the reverse of this. The onus was on me, with no one sharing the load. I found the situation to be very intense and almost claustrophobic. I suffered a lack of self-confidence and when it came to a complication with the final surgical staple, I found myself doubting my ability all the more. My anxiety in the face of being closely observed gives support to studies (Aiello and Douthitt, 2001) which have clarified earlier findings on the audience effect. It seems that close observation by passive others of activities which require improvement or further practise can reduce the quality of performance and produce feelings of apprehension.

These feelings of apprehension were likely shared with Roger as he had not had surgical staples removed before, and witnessing a student take on the role perhaps knocked his confidence further. Morse, Havens and Wilson (1997) speak of the comforting interaction-relationship model as a tool for establishing a therapeutic relationship. The model highlights some concepts for patient interaction that could benefit my practice. It is important for me when engaging with a patient prior to a procedure to talk to them and keep them calm; also if they have family members or friends present at the procedure, to include and involve them. This helps the patient to relax, and contributes to a relationship of trust. The use of individual strategies to comfort and support the patient, combining them to suit their individual needs are key to this. For example some patients may be satisfied with a preliminary explanation of a procedure. Some may wish to know more about the nurse's experience and expertise. Others may appreciate some contemporaneous phatic conversation. Still others may wish a combination of these. It is through this personalised interaction of nurse and patient that the therapeutic relationship is developed.

This process is cemented by emotional labour; the affective work involved in dealing with other peoples' feelings and regulating one's own to suit a given interaction (James, 1989). This has often been compared to acting but in the nursing context it is a way of crafting a meaningful relationship with patients within which care can take place (Mann and Cowburn, 2005). Skilled emotional labour provides socially appropriate expression of emotion which is free of disingenuous motive. Applying the comforting interaction-relationship model would help me take the focus off myself and my anxieties and refocus on the concerns of the patient by responding to the underlying reasons for his watchfulness.

The **ethical layer** of Carper's model consists of the attitudes and understandings that issue from an ethical perspective on a situation, including an awareness of moral questions and decisions.

As a nurse I will need to make ethical decisions based on my own values and level of skill. For me, I will always act to protect the patient from harm before taking responsibility for performing any procedure that could be detrimental if carried out incorrectly. This is demonstrated by the case in question, as I needed to make a decision on whether I should attempt

(continued)

(continued)

to remove the staple or refer this back to my practice teacher. Looking back both logically and ethically I made the right call, as I was able to gain experience of how to deal with these situations without putting myself or Roger at risk.

In aiming to protect the patient I was acting with beneficence, which Silva (1990) describes as four interlinked principles:

1. One should not practice evil or do harm.
2. One should prevent evil or harm.
3. One should remove evil or harm.
4. One should do good.

In this respect I was reducing the risk for the patient and operating with honest intentions. However, non-maleficence offers a more appropriate insight into this, as it recognises that it may be better not do something than to risk causing harm that outweighs the benefits (Smith, 2005). In this experience not removing the staple was safer than taking any other action on my part. I am accountable as a student nurse for my actions or lack of actions, and so the balance between beneficence and non-maleficence must be maintained appropriately to protect and empower the patient and staff involved.

The **empirical layer** is the evidence base in nursing that can be empirically verified. This can then be used to inform practice.

For most surgical wounds, staples are left in situ for 14 days as this allows the wound time to heal, while not giving it so much time that it can become sore, infected or over granulated. Moy et al. (2013) state that staples should be left in situ in large wounds for 10-14 days to reduce the risk of dehiscing and other common complications. Wound healing time can be affected by the location, size and depth of wound area; as well as genetics, lifestyle, blood supply, general health, wound infection and level of nutrition (Snowden, 1984).

Granulation tissue can continue to form within a wound or cavity even after the tissue has drawn level with the surrounding skin. This has been termed over-granulation or hyper-granulation. Hyper-granulated tissue is usually visible as a pale purple uneven mass rising above the skin level (Harris and Rolstad; 1994). The presence of such tissue prevents epithelial migration across the wound, which in turn delays wound healing (Dealey, 1999; Dunford, 1999). In the case of the final skin staple, the hyper-granulation could have occurred due to the prolonged staple placement, combined with an effective and unsupervised healing rate. This evidence finds application using the aesthetic layer of Carper's Model.

The **aesthetic layer** relates to the healthcare professional's own judgement, their ability to apply relevant evidenced based knowledge and skills to a specific situation in an individualised fashion; the content of shared knowledge and experience among professionals and patients that may or may not be found within the evidence base.

Snowden (1984) recognises that the inherent difference in healing times caused by differing factors requires the use of wound assessments and measurements as a way of individualising the wound care process. Wallenstein (2004) supports this in a study of pressure

ulcers, stating that the process of evaluating the wound allows for the assessing of treatments, and the improving of our understanding of the variables that affect the wound healing process. Giacometti et al. (2000) highlights that the symptoms of an infection include redness, swelling and pain at the site of the wound, a discharge of pus or liquid from the wound, reduced healing times, and an unpleasant smell emanating from the wound area.

The time frame for staple removal is ultimately a decision made following nursing assessment when the wound is progressing faster or slower than anticipated. Clinical judgement in this area is built on a combination of epithelisation, microbiology, pharmacology, experience of previous caring episodes, observational and olfactory skills and the patient perspective (Atkinson and Claxton, 2000). The consultant gives guidance on the average length of time the staples should be left in situ as part of the treatment plan. The nurse will decide if this should be earlier if there are signs of hyper-granulation, or later if the wound starts dehiscing or looks fragile. The nurse should also assess for signs of infection, select appropriate wound dressings and treatments, swabbing exudates for infection markers to inform prescription of medicines, working collaboratively with other disciplines where required (Dealey, 1999).

This applied combination of bodies of knowledge is at the heart of intuitive knowing. This use of evidence against experience can have a very meaningful and successful impact on service improvement. Mitchell (1994) describes intuitive knowing as a universal experience shared by everyone, and that it is the recall of knowledge without the need of evidence. In nursing practice intuition signifies knowledge recall informed by evidence to guide decisions. In this way the practitioner is permitted autonomy and flexibility in their work (Benner and Wrubel, 1989).

During this episode of care, I recognised the areas that had dehisced; also that the hyper-granulated area was red and inflamed, and was outside of my knowledge and ability as a student nurse. This self-awareness and ability to understand the limits of my practice is intuitive. It is the understanding of previous experiences and current knowledge brought together to make a safe and ethical decision.

In summary, the chance to revisit my part in communicating with patients within the context of the practical aspects of care has been invaluable. I have been helped to revisit my ability to build and maintain robust relationships through rather than despite clinical procedures by thinking on patient concerns.

Since this learning opportunity took place I have made a few key changes to my practice. I have started striking up conversation with patients about their personal interests before starting any clinical task; by doing this I put both them and myself at ease.

Even in my third year of nursing study there can still be situations that are outside my capability. Recognising that this will also be true as a graduate nurse will be essential in order for me to act ethically as well as safely and effectively. Referring to other expertise and more experienced practitioners is appropriate when faced with baffling anomalies or unexpected developments which are outside my current understanding. Continual professional development is about nothing if not about using such experiences to identify the gaps in my knowledge base. This is not only in my own best interests but also that of the patients that I care for.

Conclusion

Critical reflection is characterised by a more discriminating approach and a wider and broader search within an experience. It is an essential skill for modern nursing practice which takes account of the social, political, cultural, psychological and ethical themes which impinge upon it. Moreover, it is a process which cannot be adequately represented in a cycle. Models of critical reflection offer guidance in the shape of cues to explore the layers of knowledge in experience but their use is a means to an end rather than an end in itself. Different models will prove useful with different lived experiences.

In this chapter we have discussed critical reflection with a view to changing our practice. But once we have made room for our new knowledge how much have we changed in ourselves? The next chapter will deal with measuring change in our selves as part of perspective transformation.

6 Transformative learning

Box 6.1   Main points: Chapter 6

- Transformative learning describes a process beyond change which is merely accommodated. It describes a fundamental change in a person's values, attitudes and habits of mind to form a complete shift in perspective.
- Transformative learning takes place when the learner perceives that their previous frameworks of understanding are no longer adequate to explain reality.
- It is a painful process characterised by anxiety, anger and the mental turmoil which resembles a grieving process.
- Transformative learning is based on the ideas of Jürgen Habermas and John Mezirow. It is seen as emancipatory because it releases the learner from dependence on a teacher and from life constraints placed upon them by institutional cultural and social forces.

Introduction

This chapter builds on the principles and skills of critical reflection to introduce the notion of perspective transformation. It is entirely possible to critically reflect on some part of our practice lives advancing our learning in the process without *fundamentally changing ourselves; our personal and professional values, principles and beliefs.* We can make room for new knowledge in our lives by adjusting our behaviour without changing our values, our preferences and even our prejudices and assumptions. We will now consider transformative learning in which the learning person changes. We will be drawing primarily on the work of John Mezirow (2000; 2003) along with allied works to explore how transformational learning can take place as part of reflective practice in nursing. Once again narratives from within and without nursing life will be used to assist understanding of pertinent theory and philosophy. We will also briefly consider the contribution of neuroscience in demonstrating how we are 'wired up' for prejudice and consequently why critical reflection on experience is important and why the transformative learning process can be a difficult 'path to tread'.

Defining learning

Learning is 'any process that in living organisms leads to permanent capacity change and which is not solely due to biological maturation or ageing' (Illeris, 2007: 3). Any relationship between learning and teaching is often assumed or constructed. The idea of learning represented by a mere transfer of information from the teacher to the learner is an oversimplified misrepresentation of a complex process. The nature of this process transcends intrapersonal, corporal and social domains and is a seamless integral and mutually influential part of human development. In other words learning takes place everywhere and in every place where humans interact with their environment involving bodies as well as minds. Learning is libidinal and closely related to phylogenesis and survival. Like breathing learning is effortless. It only becomes laboured when we become conscious of it. It may be positive in the way it expands the proficiency of an individual and the contribution they make to society. While all such individuals may not be famous they live on in the minds of others through the products of their usefulness; architecture, teaching ability, humanity etc. Learning may also be negative in the shape of the regressive impact an experience may have on a person's emotional and mental wellbeing. This may give rise to correspondingly negative behaviours which form circular causality in the social and societal worlds. For example much physical violence is learned behaviour from childhood and adolescence.

Influences on knowledge acquisition

The knowledge acquisition process is influenced by the individual's genetic profile, the environment and the actions arising from the reflexivity of the individual. We may speak of a person's inherited talent for music but this is influenced by the resources made available to him, the level of encouragement he receives and the willingness to engage with music as a subject of interest with a view to acquiring mastery over it (Freeman, 1998). Moreover, all these factors are interdependent. The current controversy surrounding the identification of Attention Deficit Hyperactive Disorder (ADHD) pitched against sociological arguments claiming inappropriate medicalisation of child behaviour is an example of the nature nurture debate surrounding the relevance to learning of attention and the ability to concentrate (Illeris, 2007).

The socio-economic background of the learner is also influential on their ability to learn. Someone born in poverty will struggle against a background of poor maternal prenatal nutrition, a lack of intellectual stimulation, poor self-esteem. Haunted by calorie consuming anxiety relating to premature adult responsibility in a home life characterised by uncertainty and instabilty, such a learner will be ill at ease in a formal learning environment. Anxiety and low self-esteem will compromise their powers of concentration undermining understanding and reduced emotional intelligence excluding them from dialectical discourse. In time they may become distracted and preoccupied not least by investment in negative alternative sources of approval such as gang membership and early sexual activity (Graham and Power, 2004). Notions of assumed justice in a meritocracy are quickly discharged by such pictures of inequality in health and education. Social justice demands a system which works to widen social participation (Mezirow, 2003). A sociological perspective on knowledge acquisition sits in apposition to much habitual thinking and meaning making which apportions blame to victims of social injustice instead of recognising their need for social investment. Becoming aware of the rift of inequality in our world and its implications is an example of perspective transformation at community or societal levels. The shift in awareness is fundamental but often slow and painful because of the closely guarded deeply cherished beliefs and values that must be discharged.

The unique nature of transformational learning

While accomodative learning describes the 'accommodation of new knowledge within a preexisting framework of understanding' (accommodating or 'making room' for new knowledge), transformative learning occurs when the pre-exisiting framework of understanding is replaced with a new one. Transformative learning is sometimes called appropriation because the value base of the individual learner is changed so as to 'transform' their personality; their attitude and values in the face of thorough contemplation of the personal implications of new knowledge are irrevocably changed (Boud and Walker, 1991). Transformative learning is closely associated with the ideas of the philosopher Jürgen Habermas (Box 6.2).

Box 6.2   The ideas of Jürgen Habermas

Transformative learning is closely associated with the notion of different types of knowledge and knowing that we have visited in Chapters 3 and 5. The philosopher Jürgen Habermas (1970) argued that there were three domains of human interest inhabited by three different types of knowledge:

1.   Technical or work knowledge.
2.   Practical knowledge.
3.   Emancipatory knowledge.

Technical or work knowledge

Technical knowing is concerned with predictable rules and procedures rather like many of the clinical pathways and professional guidance discussed in Chapter 3. The rules and principles which govern such guidance are based on empirical research conducted in another setting which bears some similarity with the setting in which the guidance is being used. The assumption is that if the research were to be repeated in similar settings the results would be the same and that therefore the findings of the research can be transferred to that similar setting without fear of deviation from the original results. This thinking is governed by logical positivist ideas

(continued)

(continued)

of a particular cause having a particular effect. This type of thinking and knowing works very satisfactorily in physics, chemistry and biology where patterns are predictable but can cause problems if applied rigidly in unpredictable settings such as health and social care.

Practical knowledge

This type of knowledge is embedded in human social interaction and it thrives when all parties involved share a mutual understanding or a consensus around interpretation of what is happening. Cultural and spiritual meanings play a powerful part in this. This type of knowing and thinking is grounded in the social sciences and in psychological practices such as counselling and cognitive behavioural therapy. Practical knowledge is also used in the study of history with eye witness testimony, letters and other artefacts aiding our interpretation of past events and relationships.

Emancipatory knowledge

This way of knowing and thinking is the knowledge of self-awareness and how someone's view can be moulded by interaction with their world. The use of self, self-awareness, reflexivity, mindfulness and biographicity discussed in Chapter 1 are all forms of emancipatory knowledge. This is very much concerned with the impact of a persons life history on the way that person sees themselves. Emancipatory knowledge is also closely related to a person's perspective on their life roles and responsibilities such as parent, child, teacher, partner, employer or employee and society's expectations of them. This knowledge domain places emphasis on criticism of and liberation from social, institutional and environmental forces which limit our life choices and chances by exerting control over our lives. The term 'emancipatory' is also fitting because the learner is no longer reliant on a teacher figure in order to learn. Examples of bodies of knowledge within the emancipatory domain are feminist theory and psychotherapy. Transformative learning belongs in this domain.

A willingness to challenge oneself and explore new approaches is necessary but insuffcent on its own to navigate the full length and breadth of transformative learning. The learner must believe that all alternative courses of action are not viable. This makes transformative learning an emotionally painful and turbulent process.

Mezirow (2000: 7–8) puts it so:

> Transformative learning refers to the process by which we transform our taken for granted frames of reference (meaning perspectives, habits of mind, mindsets) to make them more inclusive, discriminating, emotionally open, capable of change and reflective so that they may generate beliefs and opinions that will prove more true or justified to guide action.

It is here that we return to the nature of meaning making referred to in the last chapter. Our way of making sense of the world by attaching concepts to phenomena means that we have a proclivity for categorical judgement to provide a feeling of secure knowledge in an unpredictable lifecourse. Stereotyping, highly selective attention, limited comprehension, projection, rationalisation, miminising or denial all play a part in construing and misconstruing through assumption because we typify individuals and events we encounter. The neural architecture of how we learn predisposes us to this (Figure 6.1). As social beings we also frequently accept and respect others as interpretative agents acting on our behalf without necessarily considering whether their methods of deduction are any more rigorous than our own. Recognising the limitations of such thinking and the absence of fixed truths is the beginning of critical reflection toward transformative learning (Mezirow, 2003).

According to Robertson (1997) transformative learning is synomynous with human development and consists of a number of phases. First of all the learner realises that the existing epistemology (or interpretive framework) which he has hitherto exposed no longer explains his experience. The process is similar to that of grief following loss. The learner exhibits anxiety and even anger and hostility in the face of such a fragmented frame of reference. Secondly, the learner searches for a fresh system of understanding which fits with the new experience. This is still a time characterised by negative emotions because of the wave of new perceptions can be overwhelming and the learner's progress toward optimum understanding seems sporadic. Acknowledging the redundant state of the former epistemology assists the learner to accept its passing. Finally the new epistemology begins to take shape as the learner understands and is able to arrange and plan his life around the implications and consequences of the new perspective. Foreknowledge of the emotional responses of a learner in the throes of transformative learning equips a teacher with the ability to empathise and assist the learner through the process.

Polanyi (1999: 143) argued that the less we guess the more we are certain and this paves the way for perspective transformation. He said:

> Because a person cannot guess what they already know, the way they see the world, the way they think and the person they are have all changed forever. Major discoveries change our interpretative framework. We cannot continue to apply former interpretative models. Discovery is therefore creative. Originality is passionate. We must leave our former selves in search of a route from problem to solution. We go there because we want to.

The idea of 'going there because we want to' is central to transformative learning and it can be illustrated in the experience of someone who successfully stops smoking after many years of contemplation (Table 6.1).

Mezirow's model of perspective transformation

Mezirow's aim is to encourage the learner to think beyond fixed long time meaning making perspectives to which they hold and to consider a range of other points of view. These alternative perspectives are informed by decompartmentalising of habitual thoughts and culturally enforced schemas as well as a consideration of external evidence. His model of perspective transformation

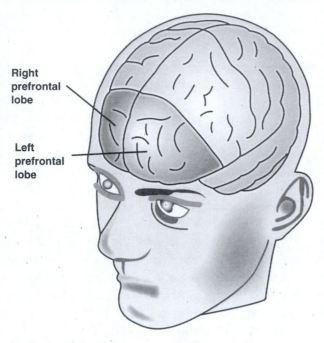

Right prefrontal lobe

Left prefrontal lobe

Prefrontal cortex

Consciousness; self-awareness and awareness of oneself in time and space, is the beginning of learning. Conscousness like the learning it facilitates is experienced in the first person and therefore all experience has personal meaning for the host. In addition the measure of personal meaning attached to information will dictate its value and the extent to which it is used. This 'sense of being' originates in the prefrontal cortex. The left frontal lobe acts as an 'encoder' giving sense to information while the right lobe manages life story themes and places them in context. It is here therefore that working memory is coupled with the decisonmaking executive (Goldberg, 2001). The prefrontal cortex has commutative links and synapses with the parietal and occipital lobes which hold images of particular events and the posterior temporal lobes which store general scenario schemas (Rose, 2006). All these structures connect with the special sensory cortices and the structures of the midbrain; notably the amygdala which processes emotions and labels, experiential concepts and the hippocampus. These structures are situated enroute between the frontal lobe and the special sensory cortices and for this reason emotions are experienced in advance of rational thought (Damassio, 1999). The importance of exploring emotions attached to an experience is therefore a crucial part of reflecting on that experience. This is possible because of 'emotion tagging' of experience so that rational and ethical thought both inform and are informed by emotions. Because of this the prefrontal cortex is able to convert information into skill and competence in the social world and intuitive thinking, knowing and doing is able to precede behaviour which is motivated by reason.

The hippocampus prioritises memories and consolidates them within the context of our episodic experience and our life story. This process which Rose (2006: 290) calls 'longterm potentiation' is consolidated when the hippocampus delivers a series of impulses or 'readout' back down the neural networks towards primary sensory regions during sleep and rest. This lends support to the theory that sleep and/or mental retiral from an experience aids learning on return to reflect on that experience.

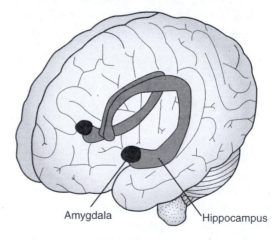

Amygdala   Hippocampus

Hippocampi and amygdala

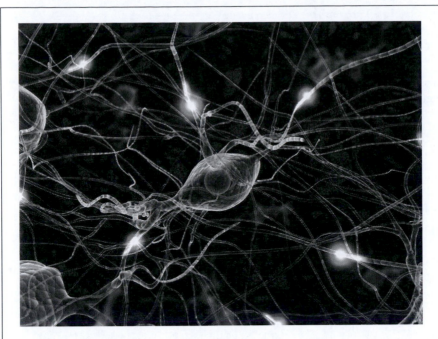

The hippocampal readout results in an engram or permanent imprint on neural tissue as the memory is stored. The more defined and integrated a memory the closer it is stored to the special sensory centres. Stimuli received from the internal environment via the thalamus and external environment via the special sensory centres are sent along cerebral neural circuits which form a multidimensional matrix forming activational associative and comparative relationships with cortical midbrain and brain stem structures (Goldberg, 2005). The structure of the neural matrix is what makes possible the specialised storage of knowledge but also the application and translation of knowledge and principles in a variety of areas instead of just one. For example mathematics can be applied to engineering and pharmacology. Ethics can be applied to law, healthcare and urban development. An associative structure is also what permits a sense of salience to guide tangential thinking and learning. Sensory experiences will stimulate memories of knowledge associated with the source of the sensory stimulus. For example a particular smell or sound may remind one of associated subject knowledge stored in memory banks. However, while the architecture and function of neural structure and circuits lends itself well to accommodative learning it does not serve the personal transformation of the individual learner well. The organisation of memories and new knowledge by the hippocampus is not involuntary. It is intentional and purposeful. As such it is managed cortically by the attention processes of the individual which in turn are fueled by the emotions, values and motives they harbour. Critical reflection is therefore necessary to attempt to unravel and identify the role that emotions, values and motives play in warping experience and learning.

Figure 6.1   Neural theories on learning

(Box 6.3) is designed to assist the learner to process an experience as they have initially perceived it in a way which is free of coercion. It provides opportunity to critique the patterns of habitual thinking and behaviour which may obscure a more enlightened view. Mezirow's model is often viewed as complex and very academic; far removed from the practical dimension of nursing life. However, as with any other model its labelled layers act as cues to guide the learner to isolate patterns of thought and behaviour which are barriers to good practice and liberate new ways of thinking, working and being.

Table 6.1 From smoker to ex-smoker to non-smoker: a narrative of transformative learning

Mere possession of knowledge may have no impact on a person's behaviour if they do not wish to change. Changing may mean relinquishing values which he cherishes and these values may override logic indefinitely. The view of cigarettes as friends and part of being 'cool' are among his taken for granted meanings.

I will never forget the day I stopped smoking. Like most people I know in my position I had been toying with the idea of ditching the 'tobacco habit' for a long time. I had been a '15–20 a day' person since I was 15 years old. I knew all the health facts. I knew about the money I would save. I'd been lectured to by my GP and had chatted with countless health promotion workers each time making promises I never kept and had no real intention of keeping. I knew I should stop for my own good and the good of others close to me. But it's not called an addiction for nothing. My relationship with cigarettes had moved on a lot since the time I had thought they made me look cool. Cigarettes were my 'friends'. They helped me feel calm when I got stressed, stopped me feeling depressed when I was lonely and most of all, they were a lovely comforting part of my day. Taking cigarettes out of my life seemed like cutting my legs off. How would I cope? Where else could I go for the sort of help or comfort they used to give me? I became very good at thinking up excuses why I could and should never stop. These thoughts alternate with irritating soliloquies about what a loser I was. So I preferred to listen to friends and workmates who also smoked and like me rationalised that 'lots of people smoke and live to a ripe old age, and anyway you have to die of something'. But I knew this was nonsense. I knew that if I went on ignoring the facts my health would suffer and prevent me enjoying all the other things I enjoyed in life.

The person wrestles with the implications of the new knowledge clinging to the hope that he need not change, together with urban myths and hearsay that support this possibility. He experiences discomfort and anxiety as part of his awkward indecision.

Then I met a wonderful girl who was very different from the women I had been with before. And yes you've guessed it: she hated smoking. The ban on smoking in public places was several weeks away. I knew this would make smoking more difficult for me and I thought to myself 'It's now or never!'

The knowledge that his habit is a threat to a new exciting relationship together with imminent change in public health legislation act as a lynchpin to engineer a corresponding change in behaviour. Behaviour change takes place because no alternative appears open to him if he is to keep his girlfriend.

This is not yet the point of transformation. The person is an ex-smoker not a non-smoker in that he grieves over his lost life and struggles to maintain his new one. It is a time of transition and the symptoms that come with the change seem overwhelming but gradually he feels more comfortable.

Relapsed thinking serves to further invalidate his old ways of thinking and doing and validate his new perspective in the shape of a stable lasting relationship and a healthy daughter he has helped to conceive. The point of transformation is reached when he hates his former way of life and has no wish to return to it.

I decided to take one day at a time. On the first day of not smoking I felt strangely confident and actually found myself bragging to friends and work colleagues that I had stopped. This confidence didn't last long. I began to develop a rash from the nicotine patches I had been prescribed by the nurse. I tell myself now I should have gone back to her but I didn't. I was astonished how constantly tired and hungry I felt throughout the days and weeks that followed. I was 'edgy' and remedies, whether nicotine chewing gum or perpetually rolling pencils and coins in my hand, brought very little respite. There were times when I could have smoked a cigarette the size of a lamp post. Along the way I gained weight and I also found out who my real friends were.

I am not sure when it started to get easier or even if 'easier' is the right word for what I experienced. I do remember that at the end of one particular day I realised that it wasn't quite as difficult as it had been. This also made me realise how far I had come and how well I had done. I somehow felt better, fitter and happier. I started to spend some of the money on myself I had saved from not smoking and that felt very good.

A year later I was a resolute ex-smoker. It was a sweltering hot day at the beginning of June and I was coming off the beach with my girlfriend. Suddenly I caught the smell of cigarette smoke blowing down wind. It was beautiful. I could have killed for a cigarette and for about half an hour I wanted to smoke again. But by the time we reached home the craving had died and I was angry with myself for how I had reasoned. That was 2 years ago. Now I am married and my wife is pregnant with our daughter. Earlier today I was leaving work and walking toward my car and it was then that I saw him; a man about my age standing smoking across the street from where my car was parked. He looked ill and prematurely old. I can't believe that I used to enjoy smoking. Now I hate the sight of it and the smell of it in a room or on peoples' clothes or skin. I have no idea how or why I ever smoked. I am now a non-smoker.

Box 6.3 Mezirow's model of perspective transformation

Reflectivity

This is the record of a disorientating dilemma. Novice reflectors call this domain 'the story' but in this model it is termed an awareness of a specific perception, meaning, behaviour or habit. This reminds us that our experience is as we perceive it to be; it is not the absolute truth.

Affective reflectivity

This domain is reserved for how you feel about what happened. Describe your feelings and link them to the parts of the experience to which they relate. Remember that our emotions are the gatekeepers of our thoughts and judgements. Exploration of our feelings often reveals our values, motives and assumptions to us.

Discriminant reflectivity

This domain is so called because it gives us the opportunity to 'discriminate' and identify our values and motives and how these shape our intentions and behaviours. To assist positive change, it is important to be able to identify the origins of these motives and values: parents, society, culture, religion. What impact did these have on what happened?

Judgemental reflectivity

The judgemental domain is concerned with isolating our goals? How would we prefer this experience to have been? What does this reveal about us? What are our habits of mind? What are our assumptions? How is such habitual thinking and assumption flawed? What needs to change to begin to achieve what we want? What is your role in this change process?

Conceptual reflectivity

This domain is the formation of a plan. How appropriate to this situation were our habitual thoughts and the approaches they moulded. Is there a pattern to our thoughts and behaviours and to what extent do they benefit or damage us? What are the advantages and disadvantages of change?

Psychic reflectivity

At this point there is a need to identify the new skills, attitudes and values needed to maintain the new perspective. The learner consolidates his new personality by replacing old habitual thought patterns with new ones rather like changing old clothes for new ones.

Theoretical reflectivity

This is the reintegration of one's life world under the new perspective. It is the bridging of the theory practice gap which represents the shift between the former self and our new self.

Leanna Hagyard (Box 6.4) uses Mezirow's Model to unravel learning from a 'near miss' experience; a narrowly avoided drug error. Leanna is shocked and confused by the realisation that drug errors are much more common than her limited practice experience had led her to believe. This previously held notion is a misleading meaning perspective. She seeks to apportion blame but finds that she has a role to play herself in the prevention of such errors. She experiences temporary anxiety as she contemplates what the ethical implications are. First she realises her lack of awareness of expert guidance. Then she comes to appreciate the role of habitualisation and potential complacency in viewing medicines administration purely as a prescription guided task.

Box 6.4   Getting to grips with drug errors

By Leanna Hagyard, third year nursing student

Considering how my habitual thoughts can impact on my practice, restricting critical evaluation of a situation, it would be beneficial to explore my experience of narrowly avoided drug error using Mezirow's Model of Reflection (Mezirow and Taylor, 2009). Mezirow's model recognises the importance of our 'habits of mind'; being aware of our own raw and unpolished thought processes allows the opportunity to enhance our points of view through self-examination and critical assessment of the habitual thinking patterns. Through successful reflection on the learned experiences, we are empowered to interpret our responses and act in an informed way, rather than upon unpolished assumptions. This therefore allows us all the freedom and confidence to become more critical in our thinking and in our practice (Hodge, 2014).

Reflectivity

My practice teacher and myself visited Mrs Beech*, a patient in receipt of palliative care whose syringe driver needed to be replenished. We also needed to review Mrs Beech's medication. In addition to the syringe driver, the patient had other forms of pain relief such as oral medication and patches, however Mrs Beech's needs for breakthrough medication had increased as a consequence of a progression in her cancer. Therefore, a decision was made to increase Mrs Beech's Diamorphine transferring the strength of her patch into the syringe driver. The suggested changes were discussed with a doctor who wrote a new prescription and we returned to Mrs Beech. Then it happened.

After drawing up the syringe I attached it to the subcutaneous line. However, just before the driver was activated, my practice teacher told me to stop as she thought she had noticed an error on the prescription. She was right. Within the syringe there was twice as much Diamorphine as was required. After recognising this, the incorrect medication was disposed of and a new prescription was sought.

(continued)

(continued)

Affective

I felt very confused. I had never been involved in a medication error before. I had never even witnessed a medication error before. I had always believed that drug errors were very rare and when they did occur it was often from a mistake which was easily recognisable and therefore easily preventable. Therefore, realising that I had been involved in such a 'near miss' with a controlled drug caused me to feel perplexed and anxious.

A medication error relates to any mistake that occurs in the prescribing, dispensing or administration of medication to a patient, regardless of whether this has had consequences for the patient or not. Each stage of the medication cycle allows an opportunity for a drug error to be recognised by the health professionals involved. Therefore, when an error occurs it indicates a crucial lack of vigilance somewhere in medicines management process (Williams, 2007).

Although the error was committed by the doctor through inaccurate prescribing, the responsibility would have been shared by my practice teacher and me. At first I solely blamed the doctor believing he should have known better but I have been given reason to reconsider this.

My practice teacher averted what would have been a calamity by double checking the prescription and consulting a conversion chart used when combining opiate medication. I was certainly glad that she had! Up until this time I'd been comfortably naive in relying on correct prescriptions and the guidance of experienced nurses. This way of thinking, if unchanged could have had dangerous implications for my future practice!

Discriminant

Although my confidence had been impeded, such an experience left me thankful for such an important lesson early in my nursing career. The near disastrous nature of the experience means that I am unlikely to forget the lesson I learned: the prevention of medication errors is challenging because it can involve practice points that are easily overlooked. For example I was not aware of the existence of a conversion chart! Some enquiry into research on medication errors to sustain increased awareness in practice is incumbent upon me.

Chergari, Manoocheri, Mohammednejad and Ehsani, (2013) point out that medication errors are among the most common health threatening mistakes which can occur in practice. Approximately 11 per cent of all prescriptions consistently involve errors of dosage (Sanders and Esmail, 2003). Errors involving morphine are among the most common (DH, 2004). Nurses play an expansive role in providing medication; approximately 40 per cent of their time in practice (Robson, 2013). This points to a greater risk of involvement in a drug error and a corresponding need for critical analysis of prescriptions for correctness and clarity and medications for appropriateness and efficacy. Nevertheless human error cannot ever be fully eradicated. Robson (2013) discusses how the majority of medication errors are founded on this with no deliberate intention to cause harm to a patient. However, deliberate abuse through inappropriate medication exists. The Shipman Enquiry (Smith, 2003) found that a family doctor had deliberately overdosed and killed over 215 patients across 24 years of his practice.

It follows therefore that as frontline coordinators of patient care nurses are accountable for ensuring at the point of administration the integrity of the medicines management process. As reflective practitioners and advocates for all patients within our care, each nurse and health professional has an obligation to ensure that their knowledge and ability to recognise a medication error is competent (NMC, 2010; 2015). This experience has exposed a gap in awareness of my accountability which I need to address.

Judgemental

There are a number of factors, which if addressed might have prevented the drug error from occurring. Firstly, my own education and awareness of resources regarding drug errors within the community would have helped.

Secondly, the role of a practice teacher is to equip their students with the knowledge and skills to succeed and provide high standards of work, an ethos that the NMC obliges each nurse to recognise and follow (NMC, 2015; RCN, 2007). The learning gleaned from a practice teacher by a student, should expand their confidence and abilities to practise autonomously and competently to ensure best care and safety for their patients. However, with expanding roles due to the promotion of home care, especially for those at end of life, is leading to further skill sets for all community nurses to possess. Correspondingly the learning needs of students in community practice settings are also expanding. So clearly drug dosage conversion methods need to be included in placement orientation in future. At the same time as an adult learner I need to resolve to be more proactive in exploring practise guidelines myself.

Prior knowledge of the conversion method wouldn't have provided me with such a harsh and memorable learning experience!

Looking at this experience from a macro perspective however, in regards to the method of conversion used by the doctor, I believe that if changes had occurred here, then there could have been a chance of the error in prescribing being avoided.

The guidance sheet used by my practice teacher to assess the conversion rates of the opioid medication was one that was used throughout her team because it was easy to understand. The doctor made his calculations using a variety of resources which unnecessarily complicated the process. So it seems that in medicines management risk may be reduced when the calculation methods used are universal across the team. Furthermore, all calculations involving opiates should be double checked and where possible the range of doses used should be limited to avoid confusion (DH, 2004).

(continued)

(continued)

Conceptual

I am now in a position to correct a range of assumptions and misconceptions. Medication errors will never be rare enough and complacency is the enemy of safety. I have also been reminded of the importance of critical thinking and mindfulness of accountability in practice. Habitualisation is avoided when the tasks of nursing are undertaken by those mindful of the art and science of nursing rather than adhering to mere task list (Benner, Tanner and Chesla, 1996). My attitude in this situation had veered a little too close to the latter. A critical questioning approach informed by best evidence serves to safeguard the patient from harm and enhance care. This does not mean that I have to be distrustful of everything and everyone. Instead I need to realise my pivotal place in front line care and the guardianship this behoves. There are two principles of ethics involved: beneficence and nonmaleficence. Beneficence is the underpinning ethical principle of nursing action; in this case the alteration of medication dose was essential to remove pain and unnecessary suffering of the patient. However, the first overriding principle is nonmaleficence checking any concerns with the prescription prior to prescribing and administration to ensure no harm occurred to the patient as consequence (Beauchamp and Childress, 2013).

Psychic

With every experience in practice a new set of learning should occur. Williams (2007) discusses how we all feel the need to shift blame onto another instead of learning and developing ourselves from our mistakes. I would much rather have blamed the doctor than be ready to consider my own part in what happened. Although it is impossible to be prepared for every situation modern practice demands a nurse who is able to use experience to bridge her theory practice gap. The incident involving the drug error has caused me never to take safe practice for granted and always be seeking ways of minimising the chance of error. No one can know everything but being open to different perspectives on a situation means being open to learning possibilities. Competence begins with practice but is sustained by reflecting on that practice.

Theoretical

I will never view drug administration in the same way again. Drug administration cannot be viewed in isolation but must be seen as part of the medicines management process. With any medication there is a risk of error occurring through either its prescribing, dispensing or administration. Knowledge and acumen alone cannot remove risk of error but risk can be managed through vigilance and awareness (Robson, 2013). Learning to step back, suspending the temptation to judge, consider different perspectives and critically evaluate roles motives and evidence will benefit not just my management of medicines but my whole practice.

Her 'discovery' that medicines administration comes under the umbrella of guardianship espoused by nurses and her realisation that administration is the final phase in a greater medicines management process means that her perspective is transformed. She will 'never view drug administration in the same way again'. Furthermore Leanna recognises the importance of a more critical questioning approach to patient drug profiles. Moreover she sees the value of 'suspending judgement' and evaluating related evidence to her whole practice. Her habitual thinking patterns are changed.

Conclusion

Transformative learning provides practitioners with the opportunity to develop personally as well as professionally in a way which mutually benefits both domains of life. It is a way of recognising the discomfort that awareness of new knowledge frameworks brings. Learners who employ transformative learning approaches are not deterred by such negative emotions but realise they signify a need to be educationally motivated. The role of reflecting on our emotional state here should not go unnoticed and implies that emotion is at the helm of our decision making. This forms the base for the discussion at the centre of the final chapter.

7

Harnessing emotion to inform clinical judgement

A new framework for reflective practice

Box 7.1   Main points: Chapter 7

- The notion of concepts rather than experiences as points for reflection opens up a new frontier in reflection and learning.
- Emotions sit at the centre of professional caring, judgement and decision making.
- Seven core emotions have been identified as having commonality across nursing practice.
- A framework composed of the concepts of anxiety, fear, anger, frustration, satisfaction, joy and sadness has potential to increase self-awareness, enhance emotional intelligence and inform practice.

Introduction

This final chapter draws on psychological and neural perspectives to examine and explore the potential for reflection in seven core emotions which have commonality across nursing practice. Essentially the notion of reflecting on concepts rather than experiences is the subject of attention. Extant literature and narratives drawn from practice are used to help explore and understand each emotion. A new framework which combines the specificity of a checklist with the freedom of intuitive thinking is introduced.

The centrality of emotion

Everything in nursing is about emotions isn't it? Reading emotion, managing emotions, using emotions, reflecting on emotions; the skills that help us control emotions and the skills that helps us use them.

(A practice educator)

A pervasive theme in this book has been the role of emotion in guiding thought and judgement. We have discussed the 'tagging' of phenomena with emotions in the prefrontal cortex to enable the conversion of knowledge to skill in the social world (Immordino-Yang and Damassio, 2007). Moreover, this forms the basis for the value of reflecting on the emotions we experience. We have stressed the importance of emotional self-awareness to the exercising of empathy (Eckroth-Bucher, 2010). We have also shown how emotional intelligence is the skilled social use of self (Goleman, 1995). In addition, we have argued that applying emotional intelligence within nursing practice means 'reading' the situated understanding of another and adjusting one's own language and behaviour accordingly (Box 7.2). In this way emotional labour grows from emotional intelligence (McQueen, 2004). This is apparent in the way a senior sister in a busy surgical ward has learned to suspend and disguise her innermost feelings in the throws of a busy shift (Box 7.3).

Box 7.2 Emotional intelligence

He is somebody that often says he doesn't like to talk about how he feels, or talk about things, so you can open up things a little bit, but then you haven't got to push him too far because that can become too difficult for him. I didn't pursue too much about what all the sadness was about because he started to block off his face and kind of close down a little bit and didn't want to give me, you know non-verbally that he didn't want to persist with it so we only stuck with it for a few minutes and then he kind of, I suppose composed himself and wasn't tearful anymore. He then started talking about related things and other things that were important, it wasn't like an avoidance, but it was taking it down a level is what I would say. My emotions in amongst all of that were just to try and keep things calm and on an even keel and to try and I suppose support him but at the same time, challenge him slightly about the way he was thinking and certainly about the way that he behaves sometimes.

(A mental health nurse consultant)

However, we have not explored how emotions can be harnessed to inform nursing judgement and practice. Yet if we accept that emotions are active at the root of judgement and decision making it ought to be possible to use them to reflect on and inform judgement and decision making.

Box 7.3 Emotional labour

I'm being interrupted all the time, I am trying to get the staff ready for handover, I am trying to support them, I've got relatives, I've got phone calls, I've got people coming in from theatre, I've got admissions and I can't get a hold of a doctor and someone is calling my name. God I swear I'm going to change my name! . . . and people say I look calm but inside I'm very anxious.

(A senior sister on an acute surgical ward)

Harnessing emotion

Relatively little work has been done in the area of harnessing emotion for professional practice. Peshkin (1988) whose work is discussed in Chapter 1 argued that subjectivity was like a 'garment that cannot be removed' in that it was a conventional wisdom which helped the researcher clarify their personal stakes in the course of their research rather than declaring them afterwards. Peshkin uncovered in himself six subjective 'I's identified arising from the emotions he experienced in the course of his work. He describes how his values, interests and the emotions related to them steered him to linger in enquiry in some areas but not in others.

Peshkin's approach was adopted in a nursing culture by Bradbury-Jones, Hughes, Murphy, Parry and Sutton (2009) in their application of Peshkin's approach to student nurse journaling. Jack (2012) has also used artwork to help students explore their emotions. All these authors report significant success in raising self-awareness. Nevertheless, their arguments while potent focus entirely on self-awareness and do not appear to consider that such reflection might be of value to anyone or anything beyond the self. No consideration is given to any commonality of emotions shared between narratives in a community of practice. Neither is there any suggestion that such commonality could be harnessed to guide judgement in situated cognition. In an eager process of using emotions to disclose the detail of the self, the value of the detail of what is provoking such emotions in the social world is overlooked.

The findings of Damassio and colleagues (1999; 2007) pertaining to the role of emotions in judgement and decision making suggest that singular emotions can be used as pivotal points for reflection. This chapter is built on the findings of a qualitative study in which thirty-three nurses in paediatrics, mental health, acute adult surgery, community and public health talked exhaustively about the emotions they experienced in practice and the causes of these emotions. Extracts from these nursing narratives feature throughout the chapter. Seven core emotions; fear, anxiety, anger, frustration, joy, sadness and satisfaction were identified as having commonality across nursing practice regardless of the specialism or experience level of the nurse. Each emotion was experienced separately but also in combination with others and often as part of a cascade leading to a more negative or more positive mood than previously experienced. The extant literature is informative as to the characteristics of each of the seven emotions.

Understanding emotions

Fear and anxiety

Historically both fear and anxiety are poorly delineated constructs in the literature but recently published authors (Orsini, Kim, Knapska and Maren, 2011; Sylvers, Lilienfeld and LaPrairie, 2011; Sauerhofer, Pamplona, Bedenk, Moll, Dawirs, von Hörsten, Wotjak and Golub, 2012) have supplied clarification on the neural and behavioural distinctions between them.

While autonomic arousal occurs during both fear and anxiety states their facilitative pathways are only partly shared. Fear is central to the 'fight or flight' process and as such is associated with the amygdaloid nuclei and increased blood flow to the right frontal lobe. However, anxiety is characterised by increased blood flow to the left frontal lobe and facilitated by the stria terminalis.

Box 7.4   Fear

Sometimes, a few occasions in the past, there has been fear, you know a child has collapsed all of a sudden and it is that adrenalin rush, 'Oh my God! What do I do now? I am frightened'. The times it has happened usually it is because of something out of your control. I think that is always a difficult thing when control gets taken away from you it makes it more, it is harder to deal with those circumstances. So fear to me, a parent or relative has been really aggressive. Or when a child has suddenly collapsed at 4am in the morning and there is no one around, you are trying your best to cope with it and the adrenalin kicks in and there is a fear of what is going to happen . . . it is almost like a feeling of panic, your heart is pounding, your mind is racing, you don't seem to be able to, you know that things are happening around you but you are actually unable to put everything in neat little boxes at that time.

(A senior sister in a paediatric unit)

Fear is accompanied by dilated pupils and orbital frontal stimulation but anxiety is not (Orsini et al., 2011; Sylvers et al., 2011). Fear is also characterised by reduced pain sensitivity due to increased levels of beta endorphins, adrenaline and noradrenalin during flight and fight responses. This is in contrast to the notion of anxiety as an emotion which results in *increased* sensitivity to external stimuli due to heightened vigilance (Sylvers et al., 2011).

Fear is present focused and manifest in the presence of a clear perceived threat and is characterised by avoidance behaviour or a rush to action. Avoidance behaviour may continue after the threat has become extinct even although this is irrational. Such a response to a 'knowing state' is regulated by the hippocampus (in the role of knowledge organiser) the amygdaloid process (in the role of arousal short circuit) and the prefrontal cortex (in the role of reasoned decision maker) (Orsini et al., 2011; Sauerhofer et al., 2012). Notice in Box 7.4. the nurse's awareness that present events

---

Box 7.5   Anxiety

I would say a little bit of anxiety because of not knowing what is going to happen and during the normal course of the day you can say, they are going to remain intubated and you don't expect anything really untoward to happen. You set your mind up, because you look after one on one, you set your mind up for, by the end of the day I want this to happen and pretty much you know it is going to happen. The child is stable, the situation is how you want it to be, but when a child is on the cusp of something, because this child wasn't intubated and that made things harder because you didn't want to re-intubate for the sake of it but you didn't want to let things go too long without intervening. So you're constantly checking in case you need to change the plan based on what you see . . . I was very worried this morning about that boy because I thought any minute now he's just going to arrest on us.

(A staff nurse in a paediatric intensive care unit)

---

are beyond her control reveal her knowledge of a clear and present danger. The mention of an 'adrenalin rush' is also consistent with the 'fight or flight' aspect of fear.

Anxiety unlike fear is future focused. It is not associated with avoidance behaviour but with anticipatory hypervigilance in the face of uncertainty. It is an emotional response to an 'unknowing state' in the shape of unresolved fear or the inability to avoid fearful stimuli. In the mind of the anxious person reality may not match expectations or a potential threat may be overestimated because of a lack of information on future options leading to indecision (Sylvers et al., 2011). The consequent stress is explained by the energy spent on framing scenarios that may never happen. The situation is governed by a 'what if' state of understanding. This is called 'catastrophising' (Meeton, Dash, Scarlet and Davey, 2012: 691). The future focused nature of anxiety is clear from the experience of the paediatric intensive care nurse in Box 7.5. The nurse compares a patient who is intubated and stable and whose care pathway is relatively predictable: you 'know pretty much what you want to happen is going to happen' with an unstable patient; one who is 'on the cusp of something'. Note the mode of hypervigilance or 'constantly checking' in the face of uncertainty and the need for readiness for a variety of scenarios: the concern that 'any moment now he is going to arrest on us'.

It is possible to experience 'anxiety with hindsight' over some past event but this is still focused on the possible future consequences of that event. Meeton et al. (2012) demonstrated that intolerance of uncertainty increases anxiety and the reduction of such uncertainty intolerance decreases anxiety. However, for nursing practice in the frontline of a social world filled with uncertainty, preparation for possibilities is a constant and anxiety is a natural companion to this.

Anger

Box 7.6   Anger

When I do eventually manage to get together to talk with people, about important team issues particularly about staffing and they say that they are going to do this and that and then nothing happens. That makes me extremely angry. It's when I am wound up. I feel provoked like I want to say something that I will later regret.

(A community nurse)

Anger is an arousal state in response to perceived threats or injustices with an identifiable source of blame. Physiological arousal is triggered in preparation for a behavioural response. Anger also increases cortisol output (Denson, 2012). Anger rumination is defined by Denson (2012: 103) as 'perseverative thinking about a personally meaningful anger-inducing event'.

In a critical review of the literature, Denson (2012) explores a multiple systems model of anger rumination with cognitive, neurobiological, affective, executive control and behavioural levels. The anger regulation effort is a tripartite mechanism: cognitive, involving suppressing anger-provoking thoughts; affective in regulating emotions; and physiological, in controlling behaviour. Attention to one aspect of self-control temporarily compromises the ability to operate another and poses a risk of aggression. Poor executive self-control can mean yielding to rumination which in turn leads to aggression. At a cognitive level a person may choose to focus on the aspects of the anger-inducing event or on the implications for the self. Cognition also governs the choice of processing mode in that an analytical approach is preoccupied with the causes and consequences of the cause of provocation. This is distinct from an experiential approach which focuses on the details of the event and the feelings it arouses. An individual's vantage perspective is also relevant to their anger experience. Viewing the root of one's anger in the first person can cause one to relive the anger-inducing incident, while viewing in the third person can induce emotional detachment. However, this latter rule applies only when taking an analytical stance. An experiential examination in the third person such as learning of injustice or persecution suffered by another may still induce anger. At a neurobiological level anger is associated with increased activity in the thalamus (the neural seat of arousal), the dorsal anterior cingulated cortex and the amygdala (associated with cognitive control) (Denson, 2012). In addition to these cortical and sub-cortical structures, anger rumination is linked to increased activity in the lateral prefrontal cortex (responsible for emotional regulation) and dorsal medial prefrontal cortex (linked to self-referential processing). At an affective level the duration and intensity of the anger experience can be greatly increased by rumination.

Although there are few differences in emotions experienced by men and women, there are differences in how those emotions are expressed. Women are more likely to conceal their anger while men are more likely to express it. A range of anger regulation strategies have been identified including verbal and non-verbal expression, leaving the situation, passive strategies such as waiting for an apology or some other change in the environment or cognitive reappraisal of the situation. In attempts at regulation, women were more likely to effectively regulate anger through distraction (Rivers, Bracket, Katulack and Salovey, 2007). Anger has been associated with more nonspecific skin conductance responses, smaller heart rate acceleration, smaller increases in stroke volume and cardiac output and larger increases in total peripheral resistance, facial temperature and finger pulse volume (Larsson, Berntson, Poehlmann, Ito and Cacioppo, 2008). The characteristics of anger are all in the experience shared by a community nurse in Box 7.6. The nurse's anger as a 'tipping point' is rooted in the failure of a manager to deliver on her promise to address a poor team staff patient ratio. The identifiable source of the resultant sense of loss means the nurse becomes 'wound up' and 'provoked' betraying the hypertensive psychosomatic features of the emotion.

Frustration

Frustration refers to the emotion experienced in the face of stemmed progress in spite of the best efforts being made. Frustration has been defined by Berkowitz (1981: 83) as a response to 'an unexpected barrier to goal attainment'. The emotion has been identified as destructive to health and productivity in the work place with Maslach, Schaufeli and Leiter (2001) identifying frustration as the penultimate phase of a downward spiralling process leading to burnout: a syndrome characterised by reduced personal achievement, emotional exhaustion and depersonalisation. Raised immunological protein S-1gA and cortisol consistent with the anticipation of stress have been shown to be present in frustrated mental states. The accompanying feeling of ill being has also been shown to lead to a range of compensatory poor health behaviours including binge eating and substance addiction. Such behaviour is compensatory in that excessive release of self-control in one area of life seeks to 'compensate' for the suppression of autonomy in another (Vansteenkiste and Ryan, 2013). Frustrated individuals will also choose between a path of rigid rule-setting, consisting of unreachably high standards to prove one's worth or oppositional defiance. The description of professional frustration by a staff nurse on a busy surgical ward (Figure 7.2) captures the essence of the emotion as it is experienced in practice. The nurse's metaphorical expression of 'being stuck in a cycle' and his talk of having the 'best laid plans' undermined by unexpected obstacles to care process are classic features of frustration.

In a study of 141 health, social care and education professionals Lewandowski (2003) found that 43 per cent of participants attributed their frustration to decreased time to care for service users. The greater the sense of isolation the less likely the worker would be to seek organisational redress due to their perception of frustration as a private matter. For 29 per cent frustration issued from the disproportionate burden of bureaucracy and the suppression of good practice by corporate rules. Lewandowski (2003: 177) proposed that the women who constitute the majority of the 'person centred working population' may have specific problems in relation to workplace frustration. She argued that the 'other focused' personal element essential for their role may undermine their ability to communicate their own needs.

Lewandowski's findings have been in part confirmed by others. A survey analysis of more than 95,000 nurses and patients by McHugh, Kutney-Lee, Cimiotti, Sloane and Aiken (2011) found a direct correlation between raised nurse dissatisfaction and low patient satisfaction.

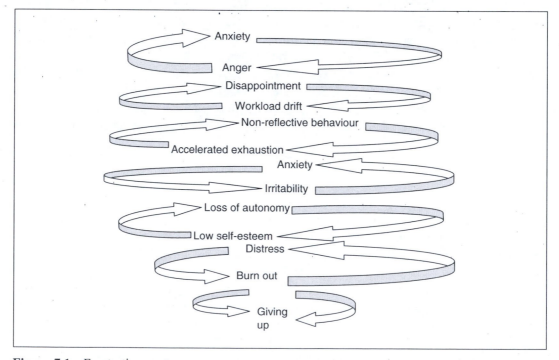

Figure 7.1   Frustration vortex

I always feel like I am always stuck in a cycle of not being able to get things done. I can't get things done I want to get done and then also on the back of that there is the ward, lack of materials, lack of drugs, having to go chasing things having to go borrowing stuff from other wards . . . the stores are always running low, we only get deliveries on Wednesday and by Friday things are already running low so it is a constant source of frustration really and then set against that you are still trying to deliver the best care that you can deliver really . . . sometimes the fax machine doesn't work or I have got to fax something over to the other wing because it is the weekend and they haven't got a pharmacy. You are trying to do a job, you are trying to do the best you can and you are thwarted by either administrative restraints, restraints of resources, staffing restraints! Every shift you have an agenda of what you want to do for your patient and then, the best laid plans of mice and men, it never happens really, there are always other things going on, there is always something out the blue.

(A staff nurse on an acute surgical ward)

Sometimes I mean kids, say you go back and you just feel it doesn't matter how much effort you put in it doesn't make a difference. So you just feel like you're just constantly going over the same ground day after day and not getting anywhere, which can make you feel quite demoralised sometimes as well because you can only keep chipping away for so long.

(A school nurse)

I think if you've put a plan into place and it is a good plan and you have tied up the loose ends and you ask somebody to follow it, it's kind of disappointing and frustrating if it doesn't happen . . . flattened maybe, I am trying to think of the physical symptoms and I can only think of disappointment being, you know dropping shoulders and the sort of, it is quite hard to articulate how that feels inside . . . sort of enthusiasm squashed out of you.

(A mental health nurse)

At one point I was getting burnt out, my colleague was too, and a number of people had gone off sick and you're still trying to provide this service to the high standard that you want to provide it to, yet you physically can't . . . therefore you feel that you're putting your patients at risk. All those things that you feel are important, like building a relationship with the patient and them believing in you and feeling that you are accessible, they all go down the drain because when there's nobody there then all that you work for, everything that you work hard trying to provide just goes.

(A district nurse)

Figure 7.2 Frustration

In view of these findings it is not surprising that workplace frustration is a predictor of intention to leave a profession. Li, Galatsch, Siegrist, Muller and Hasselhorn (2011) in a one year longitudinal study of 30,619 nurses in seven European Countries found 8.2 per cent of the total sample had expressed no intention to leave at the beginning of the study but expressed this intention at the end. Low reward exerted the strongest influence on intention to leave. Overall nurses with low rewards and high frustration were two and half times more likely to leave. The authors laid great store by the negative influence on nursing morale of working hard and receiving little or no reward in return.

Whinghter, Wang, Cunningham and Burnfield (2008) argue that avoiding goal orientation is also linked to lower levels of frustration but this option is not available to a deontological and process driven practice such as nursing. This may account for the high levels of moral distress experienced in nursing arising from ethical conflict where the ability to do what is right is far removed from the knowledge of what is right (Burston and Tuckett, 2012).

Lewandowski (2003), Li et al. (2011) and Vansteenkiste and Ryan (2013) all concur that a work environment which acknowledges and actively supports employees' difficulties and autonomous thinking forestalls frustration and boosts satisfaction.

Frustration as a lack of progress toward preset goals is therefore revealed as not debilitating by itself. Rather debilitation occurs as a result of the repeated waves of other negative emotions, disappointment, anger and sadness which parallel frustration. Conscious awareness of the root of frustration gives rise to other negative emotions such as anxiety, anger and distress in a cascade mechanism (Burston and Tuckett, 2012; Damassio, 1999). The 'drawing in' and intertwining of these powerful negative emotions in a vortex of frustration is physically, mentally and emotionally exhausting (Figure 7.1). Nursing descriptions are consistent with the pivotal point at which prolonged stress progresses to burnout as described by Maslach et al. (2001). More specifically the effort reward imbalance and it's consequences described by Li et al. (2011) are also explicit.

Satisfaction

Satisfaction developed from a combination of the Latin adjective 'satis' meaning 'enough' and the verb 'factore' meaning 'done or achieved' describes the feeling that one's desires and needs are

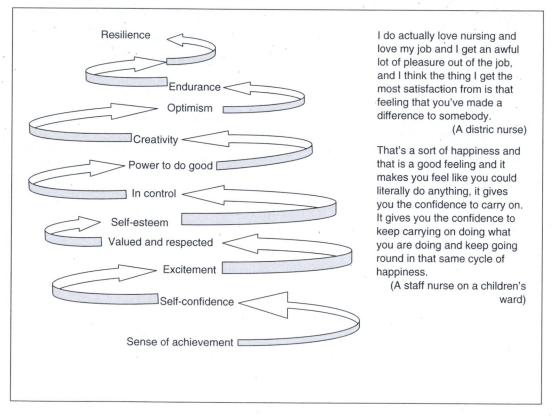

I do actually love nursing and love my job and I get an awful lot of pleasure out of the job, and I think the thing I get the most satisfaction from is that feeling that you've made a difference to somebody.
(A distric nurse)

That's a sort of happiness and that is a good feeling and it makes you feel like you could literally do anything, it gives you the confidence to carry on. It gives you the confidence to keep carrying on doing what you are doing and keep going round in that same cycle of happiness.
(A staff nurse on a children's ward)

Figure 7.3 Satisfaction

met in a way that leave no cause for complaint. The emotion is closely linked to a state of happiness, life fullness and wellbeing together with a sense of personal reward (Davern, Cummins and Stokes, 2007). Davern et al. (2007) found that there was little psychometric separation between satisfied, content and happy and concluded that these adjectives could be used interchangeably. Adams and Bond (2000: 536) agree with this in their study of satisfaction with employment. They define job satisfaction as 'the degree of positive affect towards a job or its components'. Seligman's theory of happiness as a journey through life is described in Box 7.7. Peterson, Park and Seligman (2005) showed through the use of a questionnaire completed by 845 participants that happiness and satisfaction were not consistent with an empty life but with one full of activity. However, Csikszentmihalyi (1999) cautioned that immersion solely in meaningful pursuits had limitations; a person could become so preoccupied with one particular interest so as to deprive him of other sources of satisfaction. Workaholic approaches are an example of this.

Box 7.7   Seligmans' theory of happiness

Seligman (2002) argues that we must journey through three phases of happiness before achieving genuine satisfaction:

- In the **'pleasant life'**, one learns to savour experience and reflect positively on our past with a sense of gratitude and forgiveness, accepting people and circumstances for what they are rather than for what we would wish them to be. This mind-set empowers a person to develop powerful positive emotions which enable them to look to the future with confidence and optimism.
- In the **'good life'**, the positive attitude helps one develop core personal qualities and strengths such as wisdom and courage. Seligman argues that virtuous characteristics are more powerful than talents because rather than being developed from what is inherent, they are developed through effort from nothing yet they can themselves nurture other qualities. For example, senses of humanity and justice thrive on each other. This raft of virtues equips a person to move effectively and positively in the world in a way which brings meaning to others as well as the person themselves.
- The individual is then ready to enter the most fulfilling phase: the **'meaningful life'**. Here the individual becomes influential beyond any level of personal reward and gratification they may enjoy as a result; immersing themselves in a project much larger than they are which will reach beyond their lifetime.

The importance that an individual places on a life role or roles is also significant. Perrone and Civiletto (2004) measured life role salience by participation (the amount of time spent in a particular role), commitment (the importance of a role in an individual's life world) and values expectation (the extent to which a person is able to express their values in a role). There was no variation between gender in role strain but in participation women invested more time in family and home. There was no variation for gender in the other roles. Role commitment was the only aspect of role salience which was related to role strain. High role commitment was associated with high role strain. High role strain was linked to low coping efficacy and high coping efficacy was linked to high life satisfaction. So although a high level of role salience for multiple roles can result in role strain and in distress and negative health outcomes, the authors also showed that the feeling that one is coping with multiple life roles increases life satisfaction. Cortese, Columbo and Ghislieri (2010) found that work family conflict and emotional distress were declared by all 351 respondents to their questionnaire but that job satisfaction was sustained in the presence of these factors when countered by family friendly employment policies, supportive management and supportive colleagues. These arguments sit in opposition to those of Seligman and colleagues who posit implicitly that satisfaction is chiefly a matter of personal resilience taking no account of health and social inequality or circumstance.

Enquiries into job satisfaction among nurses have been conducted both quantitatively and qualitatively. A qualitative study through the use of eight focus groups and eight face-to-face interviews with district nurses by Stuart, Jarvis and Daniel (2007) showed that the personal nature of care, the ongoing relationships with patients and the application of clinical skills and knowledge provided the greatest job satisfaction. In a review of the literature, Utrainen and Kyngas (2009) found the quality of co-worker and inter-professional relationships together with teamwork were found to be major predictors of satisfaction in the workplace. The quality of patient care being delivered; the belief among nurses that they were doing a good job and tangible visible evidence that this resulted in progress in the wellbeing of patients and their families were strong indicators of satisfaction in practice. The 'deep human connection' (2009: 1006) developed with patients arising from advocacy and the preservation of personhood and reciprocal gratitude were highly valued. These findings concur with Shaw and Degazon (2008) and Wilson and Crowe (2008) who also showed the importance to nurses of being recognised and valued by one's employing organisation. A work life balance and trustworthy relationships with colleagues were also major contributing factors to job satisfaction. These themes along with the opportunity for career development have also featured prominently in studies into job satisfaction among paediatric nurses (Wyatt and Harrison, 2010) and adult nursing in the acute hospital setting (Hayes, Bonner and Pryor, 2010).

It seems that while frustration acts like an emotional vortex drawing in a negative emotional cascade, satisfaction creates an emotional updraft which generates a positive emotional cascade (Figure 7.2). This positive cascade results in personal and professional growth and development. A sense of achievement recognised, respected and rewarded in a supportive environment promotes autonomy, swift assimilation of new knowledge and skills, creativity and innovation.

Joy

Vaillant (2008) acknowledges that joy is the least studied of all emotions yet one which holds potential for mental wellbeing. Joy has been described as a feeling of suffering removed; the essence of having been freed from captivity; of gaining or having restored to one something that may have been considered out of reach or lost. Joy is closely associated with a long sought after goal come to fruition; the release from anticipation after a sustained effort. The birth of a child or news of excellent exam results are examples of such causes for joy (Vaillant, 2008).

Causes for joy in professional practice were found by Gilat and Rosaneau (2012) in a content analysis of the written description of practice success stories by school counsellors. Professional joy was also found by Pooler, Wolfer and Freeman (2014) in interviews with twenty-six social workers who claimed to find joy in their practice. In both studies the sources of joy were less often final outcomes than significant outcome points which represented breakthroughs sitting within the process of practice. These included promoting change and empowerment, coping with resistance to change, facilitating academic success and unique learning experiences (Gilat and Rosaneau, 2012). For social workers (Pooler et al., 2014) forming relationships with other agencies and clients, having one's point of view valued, seeing the fruits of one's sustained effort, being present with people in times of distress and the contribution of work to life's purpose were all causes for joy. Pooler et al. (2014) concluded that sources of joy in professional practice should be actively sought to promote mental wellbeing and protect practitioners from burnout. The celebratory nature of joy is evident in the narrative of the children's nurse in Box 7.8. Such is the uncertainty of the outcome for the child that the nurse dare not reassure her parents in advance. However, collective joy is experienced at the news that the child's operation has been a success.

Box 7.8 Joy

You know you can't just say 'they're going to be fine' or whatever, you know because what if they're not fine you don't want to put yourself in a situation where the relative will turn around and say, 'but you told me that they're gonna be fine', but when we get the call from recovery to say that, 'oh they are in recovery, can I have a nurse?', and then I go to tell the family that the patient is in recovery – that's joy. I celebrate with the family the child is in recovery! They're awake and in recovery and they want us, and the mums leap up and they're happy and I'm happy because yes! Everything is going to be fine! And the success! So that's joy, that's the emotion that's like, 'Yes! The patient is well and they come upstairs and they're eating and drinking and peeing'.

(A staff nurse on a paediatric surgical ward)

Sadness

Sadness is an affective state associated with feelings of loss, sorrow and regret in the face of an event with no blameworthy target (Rivers, Bracket, Katulack and Salovey, 2007). Sadness is the resultant emotion from a fruitless search for a source of accountability aimed at righting a wrong. Rochman and Diamond (2008: 96) describe the experience of 'unfinished business': a stage of pointless anger and bitterness. During this phase sadness is a remedial but inaccessible state for the person. At the point at which sadness is accessed, the physiological and cognitive process is decelerated permitting a recovery period when support can be sought (Rivers et al., 2007).

The view that sadness is a powerless state lacking agency (Fischer, 1993; Tiedens, Ellsworth and Mesquita, 2000; Tiedens, 2001) has recently been challenged (Bower, 2013; Zawadzki, Warner and Shields, 2012). In a review of the literature, Bower (2013) confirms the role of sadness as a necessary and beneficial affective retreat in the aftermath of loss. Sadness was only to be damaging to judgement and wellbeing when it stretched beyond the background feeling of a few days or became more frequent to more closely resemble a longer term depressed disposition. Sadness seems to carry social benefits in that people in a sad mood were found to act with greater fairness and give greater attention to detail. Zawadzki et al. (2012) also demonstrated in a series of studies that sadness in a controlled state was a valuable resource which contributed to emotional competence and labour. Participants were repeatedly perceived as more competent when displaying managed authentic sadness in situations both related and unrelated to the emotion provoking event. Consequently both Bower (2013) and Zawadzki et al. (2012) found that resourcing present sadness and remembering past sadness states fuelled empathy.

As in the case of anger there are some gender differences in the way sadness is managed. Women are more likely to express their sadness than men who are more likely to conceal it. However, women struggle to regulate their sadness through rumination while men are more successful at regulating sadness through rumination (Rivers et al., 2007). Rivers et al. (2007) also found that sadness was commonly regulated by verbal emotional expression and seeking more information about the source of the emotion. The futility of trying to apportion blame in a cyclical situation of deprivation is immediately clear to the health visitor in Box 7.9. Her sadness envelops her sense of failure to sustain the family unit. The increased capacity for empathy in her sadness is clear as she laments over the sense of loss and devastation experienced by parents who have had their children taken permanently into care by the authorities.

Box 7.9   Sadness

I feel sadness that the parents, for whatever reason, can't adequately care for their children so they have to be removed, and I suppose its sadness as well if they've been a lot of work but actually it hasn't achieved anything. I feel sadness for the children because they, for some parents its not that they don't love their children. They just don't have the parenting capacity.

(A health visitor)

In view of the foregoing we can argue that the labelling of emotions as positive or negative is simplistic. Each emotion has its own character with positive and negative traits. This holds potential for a framework composed of emotions as points of reflection.

The potential in a common set of emotions as points for reflection

Emotions are examples of concepts. Concepts are abstract bodies of summaried ideas with senses and inferences which marshall our thoughts (Margolis and Laurence, 2000). They are the tools we use to interpret our world helping us to move virtually as well as physically within it (Pratt, 1992). Conceptual theory is derived from interaction. Intelligence can therefore be seen less as the sum of what is known than how one interacts with what one does not know or fully comprehend (Margolis and Laurence, 2000). The use of concepts as points of reflection warrants further consideration.

Emotions exist as triggers or remembrancers for wider thought. If emotions guide judgement and decision making then reflection on emotions should reveal the rationale for judgement and decision making. Comprehensive representativeness means that all seven emotions identified here hold potential as pivotal points of reflection from which all of practice life can be explored as a lived experience; providing an emotion map of nursing (Figure 7.4).

Reflecting on anxiety should prove valuable to intuitive knowing. Anxiety possesses properties of watchfulness, sensitivity and discernment in nebulous uncertain situations (Meeton et al., 2012). This holds promise for lending shape to features of practice which have previously defied definition. Such features include observed behaviours in the practice of safeguarding children and adults at risk or judgement of levels of consciousness or deterioration undetected by technical instruments in intensive care or trauma units.

The identification of threat is an important part of situational analysis. Fear will help us reflect on threats to our practice and how we might negate them. Fear supplies leverage for action and mindfulness of accountability (Sauerhöfer et al., 2012). Reflecting on anger will help us identify injustice and how we might address it. Moreover, anger will fuel advocacy (Rivers et al., 2007).

Frustration helps us identify policies, logistics, systems and behaviours which are obstructive to good practice processes and outcomes. Reflection on causes of frustration will help us act innovatively and creatively in order to move on over or around obstacles to good practice. Frustration experienced temporarily fosters greater determination to develop alternative strategies in an effort to find a way forward. This is useful when facing off powerful forces such as bureaucracy or institutional hierarchies. Frustration as a pivotal reflection point will also prove useful in the prevention of burn out (Maslach et al., 2001).

Satisfaction points to policies logistics, systems and behaviours that serve good practice and produce positive outcomes. It is a positive motivating affective force which over time musters optimism and nurtures professional skill through increased self-esteem and self-confidence. Satisfaction fosters resilience and can facilitate reframing of experience. It persists in the face of cause of more negative emotions and compensates for them. Reflecting on sources of satisfaction will help us to continually confirm our sense of fulfillment in nursing and identify what is worthy of commendation (Shaw and Degazon, 2008; Wilson and Crowe, 2008; Hayes et al., 2010; Wyatt and Harrison, 2010).

Joy issues from positive outcomes which may have seemed unlikely or impossible produced on the back of perseverance in the face of adversity. Reflecting on joy will help us to identify causes for celebration and reward in our practice. It follows that joy can pinpoint minor victories in practice which might otherwise have been eclipsed by impatience and frustration with systems and the protracted nature of the care process (Pooler et al., 2014).

Sadness reflection will help us identify causes of loss without a blame and the need for restoration. It will also help us to sustain emotional labour and empathise with patients and colleagues (Bower, 2013; Zawadzki et al., 2012).

The commonality of these emotions across nursing together with their corporate representation of the practice world suggests potential for a framework for reflection (Box 7.10). A framework for reflection on seven core emotions taken from a qualitative map of practice holds promise for

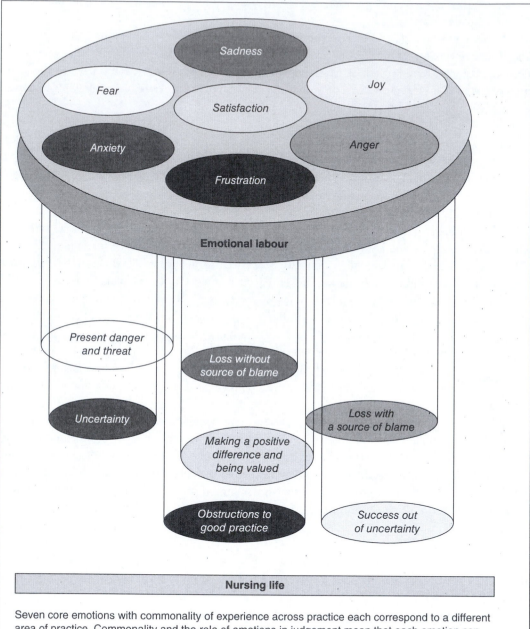

Seven core emotions with commonality of experience across practice each correspond to a different area of practice. Commonality and the role of emotions in judgement mean that each emotion can be used as a pivotal point for reflection on a different area of practice to which it relates. This type of reflection has specificity because the emotion is experienced by the user and is context specific. It has core validity because of the commonality of the emotion. The use of core emotional concepts informed by diverse narratives therefore combines the advantages of intuitive thinking with the specificity of a checklist.

Figure 7.4   The emotion map of nursing

enhancing self-awareness, emotional intelligence and informing practice. The model does not exhibit one directional signposting or 'layers' as has been the custom in past framework designs. Instead, decisions as to direction are left with the user.

Box 7.10   Frameworks and concepts

A framework is a concept map which demonstrates the relationships between concepts to reveal meaning. An ordinance survey map shows the distance and nature of terrain between one geographical location and another. A framework for counselling shows the relationship between genuineness, body language, facial expression and vocal tone.

Concepts organise our thoughts and aid our interpretation (Margolis and Laurence, 2000). However, they cannot populate a framework unless they meet certain criteria:

- Concepts must have commonality in the minds of the framework users who form a community of practice. All framework users must be able to form the same value relationships between the concepts and their practice world. For example in the world of photography light measurement, focus and shutter speed are all related concepts which will produce shared value thinking within the community of practice that is photography.
- Concepts must be repeatable and consistent in their use and application. Notice that this can also be said of the photography concepts mentioned above.
- Concepts must have economy of membership. Economy of membership is important to be useful to the user in providing pivotal thought mechanisms that are representative of diverse experience. Polanyi (1999: 78) called this the 'law of poverty' in language. If framework membership were limitless there would be no point to representativeness; a situation known as infinite regress would exist (Benner, 1984). Comprehensive representativeness means that as concepts the emotions constitute points of mental navigation for every area of praxis.

The fundamental place of emotions in judgement and decision making mean that a common set of core emotions is a powerful composite tool for practice. Such a tool should prove flexible beyond what might be expected from other prescriptive frameworks. It combines the freedom of intuitive thinking with the specificity of a checklist. Checklists are normally summaried main points gleaned from a body of research but disembodied from the real world context in which the checklist user practices. The context of practice features multiple contingencies, conditions and exit points. Consequently the checklist 'fit' with practice is often crude (Lincoln and Guba, 2000). On the other hand, emotions in the role of pivotal concepts for reflection begin with the practitioner. They exist at the seat of enquiry; the means by which people make sense of their world. Knowledge from other contexts is only admitted as relevant when deemed to fit. The seven emotions discussed in this chapter have core validity because they have commonality across the practice community. The emotions also have specificity because they are experienced by the user in their contextualised world. The

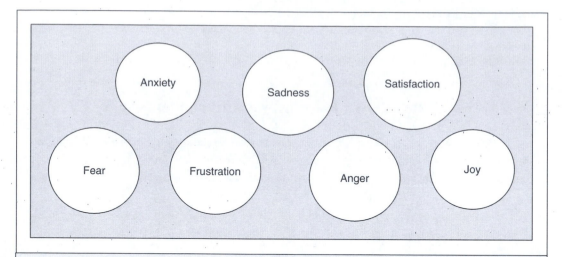

Guidelines

- The supervisee is encouraged to explore the 'menu' of emotions and choose to talk about the ones which they have experienced. The discussion should move quickly to the supervisee's identified choices.
- The supervisor and supervisee should explore together the root causes of the emotions experienced. The supervisor may use brief but repeated probing questions such as 'why?' and 'how?'.
- The supervisor and supervisee should discuss the impact on practice and agree goals arising from this discussion
- The next supervision session should begin with a review of the goals set at the last session.

The emotion framework needs to be approached and managed differently from other models of reflection. Instead of a pre-structured pathway of thought, the feeling state of the user is the constant object of enquiry. The opening question should be 'How are you?' The question simultaneously respects the personhood of the user and begins the reflection process. Socratal questioning (repeatedly asking 'why?' or 'how?' to encourage elaboration) is all that is required to maintain this process which will be informed by the situation to which the user's emotion is attached.

Figure 7.5 The emotion framework of reflective practice

symbiotic relationship between emotions and judgement mean that reflection is not restricted by the limited scope of the reflection point. Emotion as a descriptor of experience is limitless.

Conclusion

The centrality of emotion to professional caring, decision making and judgement together with the identification of seven core emotions with commonality across nursing practice form the basis for a new framework for guiding practice. The framework harnesses the positive characteristics of the anxiety, fear, anger, frustration, satisfaction, joy and sadness to inform on practice.

Conclusion

Reflection is not the holy grail of knowledge nor is it the answer to all the challenges currently facing the nursing profession. It is personalised discovery learning using an individual's own experience as the landscape. It is the way we coordinate our interpretations of different forms of knowledge giving our lives meaning and added value. Such knowledge is unlikely to be accessible in any reusable form unless a person first knows themselves well. There are many who enter nursing who will need help with this. Teachers can help by acknowledging the scale of challenge for these ones. Equally, we should understand that emotional intelligence is the difference between a nurse and a care technician. The skilled use of self preserves personhood by humanising tasks, especially those which are intrusive, embarrassing or frightening. Nurturing self-awareness will benefit every part of nursing practice, not just reflection. Discovering ourselves empowers us to maximise our strengths and seek help to address our weaknesses. Such a pathway develops resilience which helps practitioners care for themselves as well as others.

Furthermore, reflection works best when minimal control is exerted upon it and guidance is flexible and sensitive to an individual's style of learning. A uniform approach does not work because reflection is not a uniform concept. It is an organic individual one. There are certainly uniform principles but even they will be used by different people in a different order to meet the needs of learning from different experiences. Metaphors such as cycles, spirals and layers have their uses but no one metaphor will capture the shape and dynamics of such a complex process. In the same way it follows that no one model will accurately represent reflection on every experience in every person's mind. Reflection takes place in practice: the social plane of learning. So beyond the imparting of principles and process lectures on reflection have limited value.

Reflection will be best served by academic programmes when teachers adopt a partnership relationship with learners founded in the principles of adult learning. Peer learner involvement should also be encouraged. The learning support offered will need to reflect the part of the reflective process within which the learner experiences difficulty. Naturally intuitive people will sometimes feel restricted by the use of headings so they should not have them imposed upon them. Other learners will welcome the sense of focus that headings supply. Some learners will struggle to extract the salient issues from a story and they will benefit from further exploration of their feelings. Many who identify the salient issues will struggle to take these forward in any way that has meaning for their practice and they will require help with exploring the barriers to this. Moreover, anyone raised in a protected environment built on traditional values will find sociological perspectives on their experiences uncomfortable and consequently they may struggle to understand their relevance to nursing. Reflection cannot be taught as a substantive subject and there is a danger in modules designed for this purpose. In such a context reflection can be dismissed simply as a means to gain credit through formal academic assessment rather than the basis for learning meaningfully from experience throughout life.

These are difficult principles to adopt in a professional culture whose preoccupation with rituals, detailed controlling structures, rigid frameworks, pathways and measured outcomes are the norm. But sound reflective practice does not issue from such things. Sound reflective practice issues from permitting learners to think and talk about the events and episodes in professional life which matter to them and why. Sound reflective practice also means casting off the oppressive personal practices of our post modern nursing culture. This includes disowning a preoccupation with excessive criticism and self deprecation together with a reluctance to accept and commend innovative practice. Academic knowledge complements this. It does not form the basis for it. For this reason, this book ends as it began: examining the worth of emotions within the context of the therapeutic use of self.

Optimum reflection for nursing life requires the realisation that practice is best served when it is fuelled by the meaning of experience from beyond as well as within professional practice. As the narratives in this book have shown, there is much in professional practice to benefit reframing our lives as people. There is also much in our private lives that will enrich our practice.

Glossary

Amygdala or amygdaloid nucleus	The amygdala (singular) or amygdaloid process consists of two almond shaped nuclei situated bilaterally in the midbrain between the temporal lobes. The nuclei have an important role in consolidating and processing emotional memory particularly relating to fear and anxiety. In moments of crisis the amygdala is able to short circuit messages to the decision-making executive in the prefrontal cortex eliciting a faster behavioural response.
Anger	An arousal state in response to perceived threats or injustices with an identifiable source.
Anxiety	A future focused emotion arising from uncertainty with limited information on the options available. Anxiety results in increased sensitivity to external stimuli due to heightened vigilance.
Biographicity	The impact of an experience on a person's life story meaning in a fulfilling way. The person is able to reshape their life course to meet their needs and expectations. They may have cause to revaluate and reinterpret their life in view of the new perspective offered.
Catastrophising	A strategy which is sequential to anxiety in which multiple possible scenarios together with necessary responses are envisaged which may never occur. Catastrophising is governed by a 'what if' state of understanding.
Cognitive dissonance	An awareness of a clash between espoused values and behaviour.
Compassion	Awareness of suffering and pain in others which shifts the focus of our concern from ourselves and towards those ones.
Competence	Knowledge in a behavioural context; the integration of evidence based skill within everyday behaviour.
Concept translation	A principle, emotion or meaning shared between two or more contexts. The 'translation' of the concept between the contexts means that the settings that may never otherwise have been associated with one another are related.

Critical incident	A significant event or turning point valued because of the way it enables learning without a conscious search. It is sometimes called a 'light bulb' moment because of the swift inspirational way meaning is apprehended and learning is realised.
Critical reflection	The consideration of social, political, psychological, ethical and cultural influences within an experience for the purposes of meaning making and learning.
Dialectic discourse	Discussion aimed at exploring and uncovering the amount of evidence informing an opinion.
Discursive praxis	Unstructured diverse learning from experience in practice in an unplanned and unpredictable way which meanders from subject to subject.
Emotional intelligence	Social competence in perception, judgement and in relationships with others through the skilled use of self.
Emotional labour	The management of one's emotions to secure and sustain an optimum therapeutic relationship.
Empathy	The ability to represent the frame of reference of another inclusive of their emotions in one's mind.
Epistemology	The specific validated knowledge base which forms the basis for professional practice.
Fear	An emotion focused in the present. As is a response to a perceived clear and present danger it is a knowing state characterised by fight or flight; a rush to action or avoidance behaviour.
Frustration	An emotional response to the experience of an unexpected barrier to goal attainment.
Habitualisation	A state of complacency in which the expert skills integrated within experienced practice are minimised with the implication that they are common to everyone. Habitualisation in nursing arises from a lack of reflection on the complex array and use of skills in any episode of care.
Hippocampus	So called because of its resemblance to a seahorse, a structure located in the medial temporal lobe. There are two hippocampi (one in each cerebral hemisphere) responsible for the consolidation of short term memory to long term memory. Hippocampal activity increases with rest and peaks during sleep.
Intuition	Immediate apprehension through retrieval of knowledge without reasoning. The basis for intuitive knowing can be accessed through reflection.
Joy	A feeling of suffering removed; of gaining or having restored to one something that may have been considered out of reach or lost. Joy is closely associated with a long sought after goal come to fruition; the release from anticipation after a sustained effort.

Learning	Any process in living organisms which leads to permanent capacity change and which is not solely due to biological maturation or ageing.
Libidinal nature of learning	The characteristic of learning which acts as a stimulus to learn more.
Mindfulness	The ability to fully resource oneself in the present moment giving attention to the needs of the 'here and now'; discernment as to what is meaningful and deserving of personal attention in the 'moment to moment' situation.
Ontology	The nature of being. An ontological perspective is one which represents a phenomenon as it relates to a person's existence and being including their attitudes and behaviour.
Phylogenesis	The development and diversification of human knowledge and ability.
Pragmatic use of speech	The instrumental use of speech to convey subtlety in language through metaphor, hints, sarcasm, humour and irony to address the needs of the situation.
Prefrontal cortex	The part of the cerebral cortex which covers the frontal lobe. The left frontal lobe acts as an 'encoder' giving sense to information while the right lobe manages life story themes and places them in context. The medial lobe is responsible for generating confidence in judgement through a feeling of knowing. Working memory is coupled with a feeling of knowing and the decisonmaking executive. The prefrontal cortex governs social behaviour including the application of knowledge in the social world.
Propositional knowledge	Knowledge in the state of being personally owned by an individual. Propositional knowledge can take the shape of reflective narrative, eye witness statements, records and opinions.
Quasi-rationality	The combined use of different modes of judgement ranging from the harnessing of the findings of random controlled trials to intuition.
Rationalisation	The cognitive process of making something consistent or based on reason.
Reflection in action	A form of critical thinking which takes place simultaneously with practice or 'thinking on our feet'.
Reflection on action	Retrospective examination of an experience for the purpose of meaning making and learning.
Reflexivity	The ability to use an experience as a 'yard stick' for the self to promote learning and positive change.
Representational thinking	A tool for empathy in which one imagines the circumstances and emotions of another to be one's own by attempting to 'represent' them in one's mind.
Sadness	An emotion associated with loss, sorrow and regret in the face of an event with no blameworthy target.

Satisfaction	The feeling that one's desires and needs are met in a way that leave no cause for complaint and is closely linked to a state of happiness, life fullness and wellbeing together with a sense of personal reward.
Self-awareness	An understanding of ourselves which issues from a conscious knowledge of one's motives and social presentation together with how we are perceived by others.
Situated cognition	The outcome of the interaction of human interpretation with the environmental constituent(s) or object of their attention.
Social world	The domain constructed by the interpretations of the human beings who inhabit it.
Tangential thinking	Provoked cognition in a direction which is completely at odds with a current chain of thought. Thinking that is at a 'tangent' with the previous line of thinking. Tangential thinking is a central mechanism to appreciating critical incidents.
Transformational learning	The change which takes place in an individual when their pre-existing framework of understanding is replaced with another one. The process results in a fundamental change in the person's values.
Use of self	The sensitive shaping of one's personality and presence to achieve positive outcomes in relationships.

References

Aiello, J.R and Douthitt, E.A. (2001) Social Facilitation from Triplett to Economic Performance Monitoring. *Group Dynamics: Theory, Research, and Practice*, 5(3): 163–180.

Almond, P. (2001) Approaches to Decision Making and Child Protection Issues. *Community Practitioner*, 74(3): 97–100.

Appleton, J. and Cowley, S. (2004) The Guideline Contradiction: Health Visitor's Use of Formal Guidelines for Identifying and Assessing Families in Need. *International Journal of Nursing Studies*, 41(7): 785–797.

Appleton, J.V. and King, L. (1997) Intuition: A Critical Review of the Research and Rhetoric. *Journal of Advanced Nursing*, 26(1): 194–202.

Astor, P.J., Adam, M.T.P, Jähnig, C. and Seifert, S. (2013) The Joy of Winning and the Frustration of Losing: A Psychophysiological Analysis of Emotions in First-Price Sealed-Bid Auctions. *Neuroscience, Psychology, and Economics*, 6(1): 14–30.

Atkinson, T. and Claxton, G. (2000) *The Intuitive Practitioner: On the Value of Not Always Knowing What One Is Doing*. Maidenhead: Open University Press.

Attree, M. (2001) Patients' and Relatives' Experiences and Perspectives of 'Good' and 'Not so Good' Quality Care. *Journal of Advanced Nursing*, 33(4): 456–466.

Ballot, J. and Campling, P. (2011) *Intelligent Kindness: Reforming the Culture of Healthcare*. London. RCPsych Publications.

Baron-Cohen, S. (2003) *The Essential Difference*. London: Penguin.

Beauchamp, T.L. and Childress, J.F. (2013) *Principles of Biomedical Ethics*. Seventh Edition. New York: Oxford University Press.

Belsky, J. and Cassidy, J. (1994) Attachment: Theory and Practice. In: Rutter, M. and Hay, D. (Eds.), *Development through Life: A Handbook for Clinicians*. Oxford: Blackwell Science, 373–402.

Benner, P. and Tanner, C. (1987) Clinical Judgement: How Expert Nurses Use Intuition. *American Journal of Nursing*, 87(1): 23–31.

Benner, P. and Wrubel, J. (1989) On What It Is To Be a Person. In: Benner, P. and Wrubel, J. (Eds.), *The Primacy of Caring, Stress and Coping in Health and Illness*. San Francisco: Prentice Hall, 27–50.

Benner, P., Tanner, C.A. and Chesla, C.A. (1996) *Expertise in Nursing Practice, Caring, Clinical Judgement and Ethics*. New York: Springer.

Berg, L., Skott, C. and Danielson, E. (2007) Caring Relationship in a Context: Fieldwork in a Medical Ward. *International Journal of Nursing Practice*, 13(2): 100–106.

Berkowitz, L. (1981) On the Difference between Internal and External Reactions to Legitimate and Illegitimate Frustrations: A Demonstration. *Aggressive Behaviour*, 7(2): 83–96.

Billett, S., Smith, R. and Barker, M. (2005) Understanding Work, Learning and the Remaking of Cultural Practices. *Studies in Continuing Education*, 27(3): 219–237.

Blaikie, N. (1993) *Approaches to Social Inquiry*. Cambridge: Cambridge Polity Press.

Boud, D. (2010) Relocating Reflection in the Context of Practice. In: Bradbury, H., Frost, N., Kilminster, S. and Zuikas, M. (Eds.), *Beyond Reflective Practice: New Approaches to Professional Lifelong Learning*. London: Routledge, 25–36.

Boud, D., Keogh, R. and Walker, D. (1985) *Reflection: Turning Experience into Learning*. London: Kogan Page.

Bower, B. (2013) The Bright Side of Sadness. *Science News*, 184(9): 18–21.

Bradbury-Jones, C., Hughes, S.M., Murphy, W., Parry, L. and Sutton, J. (2009) A New Way of Reflecting in Nursing: The Peshkin Approach. *Journal of Advanced Nursing*, 65(11): 2485–2493.

Bredo, E. (1999) Reconstructing Educational Psychology. In: Murphy, P. (Ed.), *Learners, Learning and Assessment*. London: Sage, 23–45.

Bruner, J. (1999) *The Culture of Education*. London: Harvard University Press.

Burston, A.S. and Tuckett, A.G. (2012) Moral Distress in Nursing: Contributing Factors, Outcomes and Interventions. *Nursing Ethics*, 20(3): 312–324.

Cameron, B.L. and Mitchell, A.M. (1993) Reflective Peer Journals: Developing Authentic Nurses. *Journal of Advanced Nursing*, 18(2): 290–297.

Carlson, C.K. and Kaiser, K. (1999) Intuitive Intelligence. *Health Forum Journal*, September/October: 51–53.

Carper, B. (1978) Fundamental Patterns of Knowing. *Advances in Nursing Science*, 1(1): 13–24.

Carrol, M., Curtis, L., Higgins, A., Nichol, H., Redmond, R. and Timmins, F. (2002) Is there a Place for Reflective Practice in the Nursing Curriculum? *Clinical Effectiveness in Nursing*, 6(1): 36–41.

Chergari, M., Manoocheri, H., Mohammednejad, E. and Ehsani, S. (2013) Types and Causes of Medication Errors from a Nurses Point of View. *Iranian Journal of Nursing and Midwifery Research*, 18(3): 228–231.

Cioffi, J. (1997) Heuristics, Servants to Intuition in Clinical Decision-making. *Journal of Advanced Nursing*, 26(1): 203–208.

Clamp, C. (1980) Learning through Critical Incidents. *Nursing Times*, 76(40): 1755–1758.

Cloutier, J.D., Duncan, C. and Bailey, P.H. (2007) Locating Carper's Aesthetic Pattern of Knowing within Contemporary Evidence, Praxis and Theory. *International Journal of Nursing Educational Scholarship*, 4(1): 1–11.

Cohen, R.A. (1993) The Mutual Constraint of Memory and Attention. In: Cohen, R.A. (Ed.), *The Neuropsychology of Attention*. London: Plenum Press, 381–392.

Cowley, S. (1995) In Health Visiting, a Routine Visit Is One That Has Passed. *Journal of Advanced Nursing*, 22(2): 276–284.

Crotty, M. (1998) *The Foundations of Social Research: Meaning and Perspective in the Research Process*. London: Sage.

Crowe, M. (2000) The Nurse–Patient Relationship: A Consideration of Its Discursive Context. *Journal of Advanced Nursing*, 31(4): 962–967.

Csikszentmihalyi, M. (1999) If We Are so Rich, Why Aren't We Happy? *American Psychologist*, 54(10): 821–827.

Daniels, H. (1996) *Introduction to Vygotsky*. London: Routledge.

Damasio, A. (2000) *The Feeling of What Happens: Body and Emotion in the Making of Consciousness*. New York: Vintage.

Dashiell, J.F. (1935) Experimental Studies of the Influence of Social Situations on the Behavior of Individual Human Adults. In: Murchison, C. (Ed.), *A Handbook of Social Psychology*. Worcester: Clark University Press, 1097–1158.

Davern, M.T., Cummins, R.A. and Stokes, M.A. (2007) Subjective Wellbeing as an Affective-Cognitive Construct. *Journal of Happiness Studies*, 8(4): 429–449.

Davies, C. (1995) *Gender and the Professional Predicament in Nursing*. Buckingham: Open University Press.

Dealey, C. (1999) *The Care of Wounds: A Guide for Nurses*. Second Edition. Blackwell Science: Oxford.

Denson, T.F. (2012) The Multiple Systems Model of Angry Rumination. *Personality and Social Psychology Review*, 17(2): 103–123.

Department of Health (2004) *Building a Safer NHS for Patients: Improving Medication Safety*. London: Crown.

Dhami, M.K. and Thomson, M.E. (2012) On the Relevance of Cognitive Continuum Theory and Quasi Rationality for Understanding Management Judgement and Decision Making. *European Management Journal*, 30(4): 316–326.

Dunford, C. (1999) Hypergranulation Tissue. *Journal of Wound Care*, 8(10): 506–507.

Eckroth-Bucher, M. (2010) Self-Awareness: A Review and Analysis of a Basic Nursing Concept. *Advances in Nursing Science*, 33(4): 297–309.

English National Board (1991) *Professional Portfolio*. London: ENB.

Field, J. (2005) *Lifelong Learning and the New Educational Order*. London: Trentham Books.

Finger, M. and Asun, M. (2000) *Adult Education at the Crossroads: Learning Our Way Out*. London: Zed Books.

Finucane, T.E., Bellantoni, M. and Ouslander, J.G. (2013). Strangers in Strange Lands: The Serial Transfer of Individuals. *Journal of the American Geriatrics Society*, 61(10): 1804–1805.

Fischer, A.H. (1993) Sex Differences in Emotionality: Fact or Stereotype? *Feminism and Psychology,* 3(3): 303–318.

Flanagan, J. (1954) The Critical Incident Technique. *Psychological Bulletin,* 51(4): 327–358.

Fook, J. (2010) Reworking the 'Critical' in Critical Reflection. In: Bradbury, H., Frost, N., Kilminster, S. and Zuikas, M. (Eds.), *Beyond Reflective Practice: New Approaches to Professional Lifelong Learning*. London: Routledge, 37–51.

Francis, R. (Chair) (2013) *Report of the Mid Staffordshire NHS Foundation Trust Public Inquiry*. London: The Stationery Office.

Freeman, G. and Hughes, J. (2010). *Continuity of Care and the Patient Experience*. London: The King's Fund.

Freeman, J. (1998) Inborn Talent Exists. *Behavioral and Brain Sciences*, 21(3): 415–417.

Friere, P. (Translated by Myra Bergman Ramos) (2005) *Pedagogy of the Oppressed*. Thirtieth Anniversary Edition. London: Continuum International Publishing.

Gadamer, H.G. (1989) Truth and Method. Second Revised Edition. London: Crossroad.

Giacometti, A., Cirioni, O., Schimizzi, A.M., Del Prete, M.S., Barchiesi, F., D'Errico, M.M., Petrelli, E. and Scalise, G. (2000) Epidemiology and Microbiology of Surgical Wound Infections. *Journal of Clinical Microbiology*, 23(2): 918–922.

Gibbs, G. (1988) *Learning by Doing: A Guide to Teaching and Learning Methods*. Oxford: Oxford Polytechnic.

Giddings, L.S. (2005) Health Disparities, Social Injustice and the Culture of Nursing. *Nursing Research*, 54(5): 304–312.

Gilat, I. and Rosaneau, S. (2012) 'I Was Overcome with Joy at That Moment': Successful Experiences of School Counsellors. *British Journal of Guidance and Counselling*, 40(5): 449–463.

Gilbert, P. and Choden (2013) *Mindful Compassion: Using the Power of Mindfulness and Compassion to Transform Our Lives*. London: Robinson.

Goding, L. and Cain, P. (1999) Knowledge in Health Visiting Practice. *Nurse Education Today*, 19(4): 299–305.

Goldberg, E. (2001) *The Executive Brain: Frontal Lobes and the Civilized Mind*. New York: Oxford University Press.

Goldberg, E. (2005) *The Wisdom Paradox: How Your Mind Can Grow Stronger as Your Brain Gets Older*. New York: Gotham Books.

Goldstein, S. and Brooks, R.B. (2006) *Handbook of Resilience in Children*. London: Springer.

Goleman, D. (1995) *Emotional Intelligence: Why It Can Matter More Than IQ*. London: Bloomsbury.

Graham, H. (Ed.) (2009) *Understanding Health Inequalities*. Maidenhead: Open University Press.

Graham, H. and Power, C. (2004) *Childhood Disadvantage and Adult Health: A Lifecourse Framework.* London: Health Development Agency.

Gray, B. (2009a) The Emotional Labour in Nursing 1: Exploring the Concept. *Nursing Times*, 105(8): 26–29.

Gray, B. (2009b) Emotional Labour, Gender and Professional Stereotypes or Emotional and Physical Contact and Personal Perspectives on the Emotional Labour of Nursing. *Journal of Gender Studies*, 19(4): 349–360.

Greer, G., Pokorny, M., Clay, M.C., Brown, S. and Steele, L.L. (2010) Learner Centered Characteristics of Nurse Educators. *International Journal of Nursing Education Scholarship*, 7(1): Article 6.

Grove, S.K., Burns, N. and Gray, J.R. (2013) *The Practice of Nursing Research: Appraisal, Synthesis and Generation of Evidence.* Seventh Edition. St Louis: Elsevier Saunders.

Habermas, J. (Translated by Jeremy J. Shapiro) (1970) *Toward a Rational Society: Student Protest, Science and Politics.* London: Heinemann.

Haggerty, J.L., Reid, R.J., Freeman, G.K., Starfield, B.H., Adair, C.E. and McKendry, R. (2003) Continuity of Care: A Multidisciplinary Review. *British Medical Journal*, 327(7425): 1219–1221.

Haley, W., Larson, D., Kasl-Godley, J., Neimeyer, R. and Kwilosz, D. (2003). Roles for Psychologists in End-of-Life Care: Emerging Models of Practice. *Professional Psychology: Research and Practice, 34*(6): 626–633.

Hannigan, B. (2001) A Discussion of the Strengths and Weaknesses of 'Reflection' in Nursing Practice and Education. *Journal of Clinical Nursing*, 10: 278–273.

Haralambos, M. and Holborn, M. (2013) *Sociology Themes and Perspectives.* Eighth Edition. London: Collins.

Hargreaves, J. (1997) Using Patients: Exploring the Ethical Dimension of Reflective Practice in Nurse Education. *Journal of Advanced Nursing*, 25(2): 223–228.

Hargreaves, J. (2004) So How Do You Feel about That? Assessing Reflective Practice. *Nurse Education Today*, 24(3): 196–201.

Hargreaves, J. (2010) Voices from the Past: Professional Discourse and Reflective Practice. In: Bradbury, H., Frost, N., Kilminster, S. and Zuikas, M. (Eds.), *Beyond Reflective Practice: New Approaches to Professional Lifelong Learning.* London: Routledge, 83–95.

Harris, A. and Rolstad, B.S. (1994) Hypergranulation Tissue: A Non-Traumatic Method of Management. *Ostomy and Wound Management*, 40(5): 20–30.

Hayes, B., Bonner, A. and Pryor, J. (2010) Factors Contributing to Nurse Job Satisfaction in the Acute Hospital Setting: A Review of Recent Literature. *Journal of Nursing Management*, 18(7): 804–814.

Henderson, A. (2001) Emotional Labour and Nursing: An Underappreciated Aspect of Caring Work. *Nursing Inquiry*, 8(2): 130–138.

Hocshschild, A.R. (1983) *The Managed Heart: Commercialisation of Human Feeling.* Berkeley: University of California Press.

Hodge, S. (2014) Transformative Learning as an 'Inter-practice' Phenomenon. *Adult Education Quarterly*, 64(2): 165–181.

Howe, D., Brandon, M., Hinings, D. and Schofield, G. (1999) *Attachment Theory, Child Maltreatment and Family Support.* Basingstoke: Palgrave.

Humphreys, G.W., Riddoch, M.J., Linnell, K.J., Punt, D.J., Edwards, M.G. and Wing, A.M. (2003) Attending to What You Are Doing: Neuropsychological and Experimental Evidence for Interactions between Perception and Action. In: Humphreys and Riddoch (Eds.), *Attention in Action, Advances in Cognitive Neuroscience.* Hove: Jessica Kingsley Publishing, 3–25.

Hunynh, T., Alderson, M. and Thompson, M. (2008) Emotional Labour Underlying Caring: An Evolutionary Concept Analysis. *Journal of Advanced Nursing*, 64(2): 195–208.

Illeris, K. (2007) *How We Learn: Learning and Non-Learning in School and Beyond.* London: Routledge.

Immordino-Yang, M.H. and Damasio, A. (2007) We Feel, Therefore We Learn: The Relevance of Affective and Social Neuroscience to Education. *Mind, Brain and Education*, 1(1): 3–10.

Jack, K. (2012) 'Putting the Words "I Am Sad", Just Doesn't Quite Cut it Sometimes!': The Use of Art to Promote Emotional Awareness in Nursing Students. *Nurse Education Today*, 32(7): 811–816.

Jack, K. and Miller, E. (2008) Exploring Self-Awareness in Mental Health Practice. *Journal of Mental Health Practice*, 12(3): 31–35.

James, N. (1989) Emotional Labour: Skills and Work in the Social Regulation of Feelings: *The Sociological Review*, 37(1): 15.

Jarvis, P. (1992a) *Paradoxes of Learning: On Becoming and Individual in Society.* San Francisco: Jossey Bass.

Jarvis, P. (1992b) Reflective Practice and Nursing. *Nurse Education Today*, 12(3): 174–181.

Johns, C. (2000) *Becoming a Reflective Practitioner.* London: Blackwell Science.

Johnson, M.K. and Raye, C.L. (1998) False Memories and Confabulation. *Trends in Cognitive Sciences*, 2: 137–145.

Jones, P. (1995) Hindsight Bias in Reflective Practice: An Empirical Investigation. *Journal of Advanced Nursing*, 21(4): 783–788.

Joubert, S., Mauries, S., Barbeau, E., Ceccaldi, M. and Poncet, M. (2004) The Role of Context in Remembering Familiar Persons: Insights from Semantic Dementia. *Brain and Cognition*, 55(2): 254–261.

Kabat-Zinn, J. (1994) *Wherever You Go There You Are: Mindfulness and Meditation in Everyday Life.* New York: Hyperion.

Kawamichi, H., Tanabe, H.C., Takahasi, H.K. and Sadato, N. (2013) Activation of the Reward System during Sympathetic Concern Is Mediated by Two Types of Empathy in a Familiarity-dependent Manner. *Social Neuroscience*, 8(1): 90–100.

Kirk, T.W. (2007) Beyond Empathy: Clinical Intimacy in Nursing Practice. *Nursing Philosophy*, 8(4): 233–243.

Kitchenham, A. (2008) The Evolution of John Mezirow's Transformative Learning Theory. *Journal of Transformative Learning*, 6(2): 104–123.

Klein, L. (2001) Rigour and Intuition in Professional Life. *Ergonomics* 44(6): 579–587.

Kolb, D.A. (1984) *Experiential Learning: Experience as a Source of Learning and Development.* New Jersey: Prentice Hall.

Korthagen, F. and Vasolos, A. (2005) Levels in Reflection: Core Reflection as a Means to Enhance Professional Growth. *Teachers and Teaching: Theory and Practice*, 11(1): 47–71.

Kumar, V., Cotran, R.S. and Robbins, S.I. (2003) *Basic Pathology.* Seventh Edition. Philadephia: Saunders.

Larson, J.T., Berntson, G.G., Poehlmann, K.M., Ito, T.A. and Cacioppo, J.T. (2008) The Psychophysiology of Emotion. In: Lewis, R., Havilland-Jones, J.M. and Barratt, L.F. (Eds.), *The Handbook of Emotions.* Third Edition. New York: Guilford, 180–195.

Laurence, R.L. (2012) Intuitive Knowing and Embodied Consciousness. *New Directions for Adult and Continuing Education*, 134(1): 5–13.

Lavarack, G. (2009) *Public Health: Power, Empowerment and Professional Practice.* Second Edition. Basingstoke: Palgrave Macmillan.

Lewandowski, C.A. (2003) Organisational Factors Contributing to Worker Frustration: The Precursor to Burnout. *Journal of Sociology and Social Welfare*, 30(4): 175–185.

Li, J., Galatsch, M., Siegrist, J., Muller, B.H. and Hasselhorn, H.M. (2011) Reward Frustration at Work and Intention to Leave the Nursing Profession: Prospective Results from the European Longitudinal NEXT Study. *International Journal of Nursing Studies*, 48(5): 628–635.

Lincoln, Y.S. and Guba, E.G. (2000) The Only Generalisation Is: There Is No Generalisation. In: Gomm, Hammersley and Foster (Eds.), *Case Study Method.* London: Sage, 27–44.

Linsley, P. (2006) *Handbook of Violence and Aggression.* Milton Keynes: Radcliffe.

Livingston, G., Kelly, L. and Lewis-Holmes, E. (2014) Non-pharmacological Interventions for Agitation in Dementia: Systematic Review of Randomised Controlled Trials. *British Journal of Psychiatry*, 205(6): 436–442.

Lotman, Y. (1990) The Notion of Boundary. In: *The Universe of the Mind: A Semiotic Theory of Culture.* London: I.B. Tauris, 131–142.

Luft, J. and Ingham, H. (1955) The Johari Window: A Graphic Model for Interpersonal Relations. California: University of California.

Maclaren, J. (2002) Reflecting on Your Expert Practice. *Nursing Times*, 98:(9), 38–39.

Malloch, K. (2000) Nurse Patient Relationships: Essential Skills for Expert Nursing Practice. *Creative Nursing*, 4(4): 12–13.

Mann, S., and Cowburn, J. (2005) Emotional Labour and Stress within Mental Health Nursing. *Journal of Psychiatric and Mental Health Nursing*, 12(2): 154–162.

Margolis, E. and Laurence, S. (2000) Concepts in Cognitive Science. In: Margolis, E. and Laurence, S. (Eds.), *Concepts, Core Readings*. Second Edition. Boston: Massachusetts Institute of Technology, 3–81.

Marmot, M. and Wilkinson, R. (Eds.) (2006) *Social Determinants of Health*. Second Edition. Oxford: Oxford University Press.

Maslach, C., Schaufeli, W. and Leiter, M.P. (2001) Job Burnout. *Annual Review of Psychology*, 52(1): 397–422.

Mazhindu, D.M. (2003) Ideal Nurses: The Social Construction of Emotional Labour. *European Journal of Psychotherapy, Counselling and Health*, 6(3): 243–262.

McCormack, B. (2003) A Conceptual Framework for Person-centred Practice with Older People. *International Journal of Nursing Practice*, 9(3): 202–209.

McHugh, M.D., Kutney-Lee, A., Cimiotti, J.P., Sloane, D.M. and Aiken, L.H. (2011) Nurses' Widespread Job Dissatisfaction, Burnout, and Frustration with Health Benefits Signal Problems for Patient Care. *Health Affairs,* 30(2): 202–210.

McKinnon, J. (2011) The Nurse–Patient Relationship. In: Linsley, P., Kane, R. and Owen, S. (Eds.), *Nursing for Public Health: Promotion, Principles, and Practice*. Oxford: Oxford University Press, 64–74.

McKinnon, J. (2014) Transformational Learning. In: Lynsley, P., Hurley, J and van der Zwan, R. (Eds.), *Emotions in Educational Settings*. Brisbane: Oxford Global Press, 111–132.

McQueen, A.C.H. (2004) Emotional Intelligence in Nursing Work. *Journal of Advanced Nursing*, 47(1): 101–108.

Meeten, F., Dash, S.R., Scarlet, A.L.S. and Davey, G.L.C. (2012) Investigating the Effect of Intolerance of Uncertainty on Castastrophic Worrying and Mood. *Behaviour Research and Therapy*, 50(11): 690–698.

Messam, K. and Pettifer, A. (2009). Understanding Best Practice within Nurse Intershift Handover: What Suits Palliative Care? *International Journal of Palliative Nursing*, 15(4): 190–197.

Mezirow, J. (2000) Learning to Think Like an Adult: Core Conceptions of Transformative Theory. In: Mezirow, J. (Ed.), *Learning as Transformation: Critical Perspectives and Theory in Progress*. San Francisco: Jossey Bass, 7–8.

Mezirow, J. (2003) Transformative Learning as Discourse. *Journal of Transformative Education*, 1(1): 58–63.

Mezirow, J. and Taylor, E.W. (2009). *Transformative Learning in Practice: Insights from Community, Workplace, and Higher Education*. San Francisco: Jossey-Bass.

Mitchell, G. (1994) Intuitive Knowing: Exposing a Myth in Theory Development. *Nursing Science Quarterly*, 7(1): 2–3.

Modirrousta, M. and Fellows, L.K. (2008) Media Prefrontal Cortex Plays a Critical and Selective Role in Feeling and Knowing Meta-Memory Judgements. *Neuropsychologia*, 46(12): 2958–2965.

Morse, J.M., Havens, G.A. and Wilson, S. (1997) The Comforting Interaction: Developing a Model of Nurse-Patient Relationship. *Scholarly Inquiry for Nursing Practice*, 11(4): 321.43–345.7.

Motahari, M. (2008) The Hermeneutical Circle or the Hermeneutical Spiral? *International Journal of Humanities*, 15(2): 99–111.

Moy, R.L., Waldman, B. and Hein, D.W. (2013) A Review of Sutures and Suturing Techniques. *The Journal of Dermatologic Surgery and Oncology*, 18(9): 785–795.

Mulhall, A. (1998) Nursing, Research and the Evidence. *Evidence Based Nursing*, 1(1): 4–6.

Murphy, D. (2011) The Liverpool Care Pathway Provides Clarity and Focus: Communication, Care and Compassion Come from You [Editorial]. *International Journal of Palliative Nursing*, 17(11): 529.

Negus, D. (2005) *Leg Ulcers: Diagnosis and Management*. Third Edition. Oxford: Taylor and Francis.

Nelms, T.P. and Lane, E.B. (1999) Women's Ways of Knowing and Critical Thinking. *Professional Nurse*, 15(3): 179–186.

Niedenthal, P.M., Krauth-Gruber, S. and Ric, F. (2006) *Psychology of Emotion, Interpersonal, Experiential, and Cognitive Approaches*. Hove: Psychology Press.

Nursing and Midwifery Council of United Kingdom (2010) *Standards for Medicines Management*. London: NMC.

Nursing and Midwifery Council of United Kingdom (2015) *The Code: Standards of Conduct, Performance and Ethics for Nurses and Midwives*. London: NMC.

Oleson, H.S. (1989) *Adult Education and Everyday Life*. Roskilde: The Adult Education Research Group, Roskilde University.

Orsini, C.A., Kim, J.H., Knapska, E. and Maren, S. (2011) Hippocampal and Prefrontal Projections to the Basal Amygdala Mediate Contextual Regulation of Fear after Extinction. *Journal of Neuroscience*, 31(47): 17269–17277.

Pask, E. (1995) Trust: An Essential Component of Nursing Practice – Implications for Nurse Education. *Nurse Education Today*, 15(3): 190–195.

Paterson, B. (1995) Developing and Maintaining Reflection in Clinical Journals. *Nurse Education Today*, 15(3): 211–220.

Peate, I. (2007) *Becoming a Nurse in the 21st Century*. Chichester: John Wiley and Sons Ltd.

Pennington, N. and Hastie, R. (1986) Evidence Evaluation in Complex Decision Making. *Journal of Personality and Social Psychology*, 51(2): 242–258.

Pennington, N. and Hastie, R. (1988) Explanation-Based Decision Making: Effects of Memory Structure on Judgement. *Journal of Experimental Psychology: Learning, Memory, Cognition*, 14(3): 521–533.

Perrone, K.L., Civiletto, C.L. (2004) The Impact of Life Role Salience on Life Satisfaction. *Journal of Employment Counselling*, 41(3): 105–117.

Peshkin, A. (1988) In Search of Subjectivity – One's Own. *Educational Researcher*, 17(7): 17–21.

Peterson, C., Park, M. and Seligman, M.E.P. (2005) Orientations to Happiness and Life Satisfaction: The Full Life versus the Empty Life. *Journal of Happiness Studies*, 6(1): 25–41.

Polanyi, M. (1998) *Personal Knowledge: Towards a Post Critical Philosophy*. London: Routledge.

Pooler, D.K., Wolfer, T.A. and Freeman, M.L. (2014) Finding Joy in Social Work: Interpersonal Sources. *Family in Society*, 95(1): 34–42.

Pratt, D.D. (1992) Conceptions of Teaching. *Adult Education Quarterley*, 42(4): 203–220.

Preston, M. (2007) The Liverpool Care Pathway for the Dying Patient: A Guide to Implementation. *End of Life Care*, 1(1): 61–68.

Pronin, E. and Kugler, M. (2006) Valuing Thoughts, Ignoring Behaviour: The Introspection Illusion as a Source of the Bias Blind Spot. *Journal of Experimental Social Psychology*, 43(4): 565–578.

Reid, B. (1993) 'But We're Doing it Already?' Exploring a Response to the Concept of Reflective Practice in Order to Improve Its Facilitation. *Nurse Education Today*, 13(4): 305–209.

Rich, A. and Parker, D.L. (1995) Reflection and Critical Incident Analysis: Ethical and Moral Implications of Their Use within Nursing and Midwifery Education. *Journal of Advanced Nursing*, 22(6): 1050–1057.

Richardson, G. and Maltby, H. (1995) Reflection-on-Practice: Enhancing Student Learning. *Journal of Advanced Nursing*, 22(2): 235–242.

Rigg, C. and Trehan, K. (2008) Critical Reflection: Is It Just Too Difficult? *Journal of European Industrial Training*, 32(5): 374–384.

Riley-Doucet, C. and Wilson, S. (1997) A Three Step Method of Self-Reflection Using Reflective Journal Writing. *Journal of Advanced Nursing*, 25(5): 964–968.

Rivers, S.E., Bracket, M.A., Katulack, N.A. and Salovey, P. (2007) Regulating Anger and Sadness: An Exploration of Discrete Emotions in Emotional Regulation. *Journal of Happiness Studies*, 8(3): 393–427.

Robbins, D. (2001) *Vygotsky's Psychology-philosophy: A Metaphor for Language Theory and Learning*. London: Kluwer Academic/Plenum Publishers.

Robertson, D.L. (1997) Transformative Learning and Transition Theory: Toward Developing the Ability to Facilitate Insight. *Journal on Excellence in College Teaching,* 8(1): 105–125.

Robson, W. (2013) Prescribing Errors: Taking the Human Factor into Account. *Nurse Prescribing,* 11(9): 455–458.

Rochman, D. and Diamond, G.M. (2008) From Unresolved Anger to Sadness: Identifying Physiological Correlates. *Journal of Counselling Psychology,* 55(1): 96–105.

Rogers, C. (1994) *Freedom to Learn.* Third Edition. New York: Macmillan College.

Rose, D. (2006) *Consciousness, Philosophical, Psychological and Neural Theories.* Oxford: Oxford University Press.

Royal College of Nursing (2005) *Bullying and Harassment at Work: A Good Practice Guide for RCN Negotiators and Health Care Managers.* London: RCN.

Royal College of Nursing (2007) *Guidance for Mentors of Nursing Students and Midwives. An RCN Toolkit.* Second Edition. London: RCN.

Saint-Exupery, A. (2000) *The Little Prince.* Florida: Harcourt Inc.

Sanders, J. and Esmail, A. (2003) The Frequency and Nature of Medical Error in Primary Care: Understanding the Diversity Across Studies. *Family Practice,* 20(3): 231–236.

Sauerhöfer, E., Pamplona, F.A., Bedenk, B., Moll, G.H., Dawirs, R.R., von Hörsten, S., Wotjak, C. and Golub, Y. (2012) Generalization of Contextual Fear Depends on Associative Rather than Non-associative Memory Components. *Behavioural Brain Research,* 233(2): 483–493.

Scheffer, B.K. and Rubenfeld, G. (1999) Thinking Mode Classification. In: Scheffer, B.K. and Rubenfeld, G. *Critical Thinking in Nursing: An Interactive Approach.* Second Edition. London: Lippincott, Williams and Wilkins, 1: 3–29.

Schon, D.A. (1987) *The Reflective Practitioner: How Professionals Think in Action.* New York: Basic Books.

Scott, P.A. (2000) Emotion, Moral Perception and Nursing Practice. *Nursing Philosophy,* 1(1): 123–133.

Seedhouse, D. (2008) *Ethics: The Heart of Healthcare.* Third Edition. Chichester: John Wiley and Sons Ltd.

Seligman, M.E.P (2002) *Authentic Happiness: Using the New Positive Psychology to Realize Your Potential for Lasting Fulfillment.* New York: Free Press.

Shaw, H.K. and Degazon, C. (2008) Integrating the Core Professional Values of Nursing: A Profession, Not Just a Career. *Journal of Cultural Diversity,* 15(1): 44–50.

Silva, M.C. (1990) *Ethical Decision Making in Nursing Administration.* Norwalk: Appleton & Lange.

Simon, D.A., Dix, F.P., McCollum, C.N. (2004) The Management of Venous Leg Ulcers. *British Medical Journal,* 328(7452): 1358–1362.

Smith, C.M. (2005) Origin and Uses of Primum Non Nocere: Above All, Do No Harm! *The Journal of Clinical Pharmacology,* 45(4): 371–377.

Smith, J. (2003) *The Shipman Inquiry. 3rd Report. Death Certification and the Investigation of Deaths by Coroners.* Norwich: Crown Publishers.

Snowden, J. (1984) Wound Closure: An Analysis of the Relative Contributions of Contraction and Epithilialization (sic). *Journal of Surgical Research,* 37(6): 453–463.

Solms, M. and Turnbull, O. (2002) *The Brain and the Inner World: An Introduction to the Neuroscience of Subjective Experience.* London: Karnac.

Stake, R. (2000) Case Study Method of Social Inquiry. In: Gomm, Hammersley and Foster (Eds.), *Case Study Method.* London: Sage, 19–26.

Standing, M. (2008) Clinical Judgement and Decision Making in Nursing: Nine Modes of Practice in a Revised Cognitive Continuum. *Journal of Advanced Nursing,* 62(1): 124–134.

Standish, P., Smeyers, P. and Smith, R. (2006) *The Therapy of Education: Philosophy, Happiness and Personal Growth.* Basingstoke: Palgrave Macmillan.

Stayt, L.C. (2008) Death, Empathy and Self-Preservation: The Emotional Labour of Caring for Families of the Critically Ill in Adult Intensive Care. *Journal of Clinical Nursing,* 18(9): 1267–1275.

Stickley, T., Freshwater, D. (2006) The Art of Listening in the Therapeutic Relationship. *Mental Health Practice,* 9(5): 12–18.

Strauss, A. and Corbin, J. (1990) *Basics of Qualitative Research, Grounded Theory Procedures and Techniques*. London: Sage.

Stuart, E.H., Jarvis, A. and Daniel, K. (2007) A Ward without Walls? District Nurses Perceptions of their Workload, Management Priorities and Job Satisfaction. *Journal of Clinical Nursing*, 17(22): 3012–3020.

Swann, J.I. (2013) Dementia and Reminiscence: Not Just a Focus on the Past. *British Journal of Healthcare Assistants*, 7(12): 614–617.

Sylvers, P., Lilienfeld, S.O. and LaPrairie, J.L. (2011) Differences between Trait Fear and Trait Anxiety: Implications for Psychopathology. *Clinical Psychology Review*, 31: 122–137.

Talbot, J. (2012) *Work Based Learning e-Journal International*, 2(2) http://wblearning-ejournal.com/currentIssue/E4002.pdf [Accessed 20 November 2012].

Theodosius, C. (2008) *Emotional Labour in Health Care: The Unmanaged Heart of Nursing*. London: Routledge.

Tiedens, L.Z. (2001) Anger and Advancement versus Sadness and Subjugation: The Effect of Negative Emotion Expressions on Social Status Conferral. *Journal of Personality and Social Psychology*, 80(1): 86–94.

Tiedens, L.Z., Ellsworth, P.C. and Mesquita, B. (2000). Stereotypes about Sentiments and Status: Emotional Expectations for High and Low Status Group Members. *Personality and Social Psychology Bulletin*, 26(5): 560–575.

Tortora, G. and Derrickson, B. (2006) *Principles of Anatomy and Physiology*. Hoboken: John Wiley and Sons Ltd.

Travis, L.E. (1925) The Effect of a Small Audience upon Eye–Hand Coordination. *Journal of Abnormal and Social Psychology*, 20(2): 142.

Tripp, D. (1993) *Critical Incidents in Teaching, Developing Professional Judgement*. London: Routledge.

Tulving, E. and Schacter, D.L. (1990) Priming and Human Memory Systems. *Science*, 247(4940): 301–306.

UKCC (1999) *The PREP Handbook: Post-Registration Education and Practice*. London: UKCC.

Utrainen, K. and Kyngas, H. (2009) Hospital Nurses' Job Satisfaction: A Literature Review. *Journal of Nursing Management*. 17(8): 1002–1010.

Vaillant, G. (2008) *Spiritual Evolution: A Scientific Defense of Faith*. New York: Broadway Books.

Vansteenkiste, M. and Ryan, R.M. (2013) On Psychological Growth and Vulnerability: Basic Psychological Need Satisfaction and Need Frustration as a Unifying Principle. *Journal of Psychotherapy Integration*, 23(3): 263–280.

Velleman, R., Copello, A. and Maslin, J. (1998) *Living with Drink: Women Who Live with Problem Drinkers*. Harlow: Longman.

Vrij, A. (2000) *Detecting Lies and Deceit: The Psychology of Lying and the Implications for Professional Practice*. Chichester: John Wiley and Sons Ltd.

Wallenstein, S. (2004) Statistical Analysis of Wound Healing Rates for Pressure Ulcers: *The American Journal of Surgery*, 188(1): 73–78.

Welland, S.J. and Bethune E. (1996) Reflective Journal Writing in Nurse Education: Whose Interests Does It Serve? *Journal of Advanced Nursing*, 24(5): 1077–1082.

White, L. (2014) Mindfulness in Nursing: An Evolutionary Concept Analysis. *Journal of Advanced Nursing*, 70(2): 282–294.

Wilde, M.H. and Garvin, S. (2007) A Concept Analysis of Self-monitoring. *Journal of Advanced Nursing*, 57(3): 339–350.

Wilkinson, J. (1999) Implementing Reflective Practice. *Nursing Standard*. 13(21): 36–40.

Williams, A. (2001) A Study of Practising Nurses' Perceptions and Experiences of Intimacy within the Nurse–Patient Relationship. *Journal of Advanced Nursing*, 35(2): 188–196.

Williams, D. (2007) Medication Errors. *Journal of Royal College of Physicians of Edinburgh*, 37(3): 343–346.

Wilson, B. and Crowe, M. (2008) Maintaining Equilibrium: A Theory of Job Satisfaction for Community Mental Health Nurses. *Journal of Psychiatric and Mental Health Nursing*, 15(10): 816–822.

Wyatt, J. and Harrison, M. (2010) Certified Pediatric Nurses Perceptions of Job Satisfaction. *Pediatric Nursing*, 36(4): 205–208.

Zammuner, V.L. and Galli, C. (2005) Wellbeing: Causes and Consequences of Emotion Regulation in Work Settings. *International Review of Psychiatry*, 17(5): 355–364.

Zawadzki, M.J., Warner, L.R. and Shields, S.A. (2013) Sadness Is Believed to Signal Competence When Displayed with Passionate Restraint. *Social Psychology*, 44(3): 219–230.

Zembylas, M. (2005) Three Perspectives on Linking the Cognitive and the Emotional in Science Learning: Conceptual Change, Socio-Constructivism and Post-Structuralism. *Studies in Science Education*, 41: 91–116.

Index